IN THE COMPANY OF
ANGELS

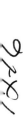

Pamela Jean Lyman

IN THE COMPANY OF

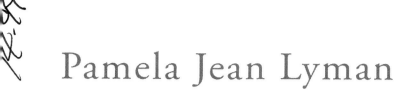

a compilation of stories and poems
on Angelman Syndrome,
by those who know it best

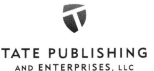

TATE PUBLISHING
AND ENTERPRISES, LLC

Scripture quotations marked "NIV" are taken from the *Holy Bible, New International Version* ®, Copyright © 1973, 1978, 1984 by International Bible Society. Used by permission of Zondervan Publishing House. All rights reserved.

Scripture quotations marked "MSG" are taken from *The Message*, Copyright © 1993, 1994, 1995, 1996, 2000, 2001, 2002. Used by permission of NavPress Publishing Group. All rights reserved.

Scripture quotations marked "CEV" are from the *Holy Bible; Contemporary English Version,* Copyright © 1995, Barclay M. Newman, ed., American Bible Society. Used by permission. All rights reserved.

The opinions expressed by the author are not necessarily those of Tate Publishing, LLC.

Published by Tate Publishing & Enterprises, LLC
127 E. Trade Center Terrace | Mustang, Oklahoma 73064 USA
1.888.361.9473 | www.tatepublishing.com

Tate Publishing is committed to excellence in the publishing industry. The company reflects the philosophy established by the founders, based on Psalm 68:11,
"The Lord gave the word and great was the company of those who published it."

Book design copyright © 2012 by Tate Publishing, LLC. All rights reserved.
Cover design by Matias Alasagas
Interior design by Joana Quilantang

Published in the United States of America

ISBN:978-1-62147-564-4
1. Health & Fitness / Diseases / Genetic
2. Family & Relationship / Children with Special Needs
12.11.05

3 4766 00468557 0

DEDICATION

This book is dedicated to
my supportive and loving husband, Matt,
who helps me find the humor in the daily grind,
and to our four incredible boys,
Ben, Conrad, George and Wilson.

TABLE OF CONTENTS

PREFACE

Angelman syndrome (often abbreviated AS), is a severe neurological disorder characterized by profound developmental delays, problems with motor coordination (ataxia) and balance, and epilepsy. Individuals with AS do not develop functional speech. The seizure disorder in individuals with Angelman syndrome can be difficult to treat. Feeding disorders in infancy are common, and some persist throughout childhood. Sleeping difficulties are commonly noted in individuals with Angelman syndrome. AS affects all races and both genders equally.

Individuals with Angelman syndrome tend to have a happy demeanor, characterized by frequent laughing, smiling, and excitability. Many individuals with Angelman syndrome are attracted to water and take great pleasure in activities like swimming and bathing. People living with AS require lifelong care, intense therapies to help develop functional skills and improve their quality of life, and close medical supervision, often involving multiple medical interventions. Angelman syndrome may be misdiagnosed since other syndromes have similar characteristics.

Angelman syndrome is a genetic-based disorder resulting from the loss of function of the Ube3a gene in the brain. Loss of Ube3a prevents neurons from functioning correctly, leading to deficits in learning and memory. Importantly, loss of UBE3A does not appear to affect neuronal development, indicating that neurons could function normally if UBE3A function is restored.

(Taken with permission from the excellent website www.cureangelman.org)

FOREWORD

After the diagnosis of our son Conrad, I immediately began looking for books on Angelman syndrome. I wanted to read someone else's story about how they were raising a child with Angelman Syndrome. I wanted to know that one could have a normal life while having a disabled child. I wanted to know how the siblings, grandparents, aunts, uncles, cousins, and friends of a disabled child handled this experience. I needed to know that my new life was manageable and doable and could be somewhat *normal.* Mostly, I hungered for the reassurance that *I* could mother a child with a disability—one, I had just learned, who would never (maybe), say any words, might never be potty-trained, may always live at home, and would be severely handicapped for his entire life. I had to hear other people's stories. I had to understand how others had done this so that I could know that I could do it too.

I searched and searched for the right book, but Angelman syndrome is rare—there were very few resources to choose from. Finally, after some prompting from my mother-in-law (whose motto is, "You can do hard things"), I set out to write the book I was looking for.

With the help of the Canadian Angelman Syndrome Society (CASS), the Angelman Syndrome Foundation (ASF), and the Foundation for Angelman Syndrome Therapeutics (FAST), I started collecting amazing stories, poems, and pictures from all around the world from people intimately connected to this rare genetic disorder. As the accounts from beloved families and friends came pouring in, I was often overcome with emotion. These were words and images enveloped in love...sealed with joy, grief, humor, and resolve. I have laughed and wept with these Angel friends who have shared their lives with me. It has been an honor to compile their stories.

It is my hope and my prayer that this book helps someone else know that they are not alone in the struggle to raise a child with a disability, even one as rare as Angelman syndrome. I hope that all who read these stories will emerge, as I have, enlightened and empowered.

I have gained such strength from reading these accounts of people living my similar life. I now have the courage and resolve to move forward while raising a child with a disability. Sometimes the task is daunting and the path unclear as I reach challenges with Conrad that I feel ill-equipped to handle. Knowing that there are others out there facing the same difficulties makes the struggles easier to bear.

Each day, in spite of the challenges, I count myself fortunate to be a part of an extraordinary group of Angel mothers, fathers, siblings, grandparents, cousins, friends, and care providers.

I thank them—and all the Angels of this world—from the bottom of my heart.

PART ONE: MY STORY

CONRADICAL

By Pamela B. Lyman
Mother to Conrad

Conrad Jefferson Lyman was born late in the evening of March 30, 2002. As I sat on the couch waiting for my mother-in-law to arrive to take care of our older son, Ben, I began to cry. I was about to enter a new chapter in my life with two children, and I wasn't sure I was ready. Ben and I had so much fun together, and I was afraid that I might not love this new baby as much as him. I had an inclination that something was going to be different with this child. The feeling made me anxious. I wasn't sure if it was the kind of anxiety to fear or to embrace.

Even though my labor was long and exhaustive, there was a sort of peace that resonated in the room right before Conrad entered the world. The anxiety that I had felt earlier in the day was replaced with joy. As soon as I laid eyes on him I fell madly in love. I knew the instant he was placed in my arms that he was special, and that God had entrusted me, us, with one of his most precious spirits.

As we were driving home from the hospital with Conrad tucked neatly in his car seat, I watched him closely and tried to figure out what made him special in a way different from our first child.

From the moment we brought him through our door the spirit of our home was different. He looked so wise for such a tiny being. I craved being around him and feeling of his spirit.

Soon I began to realize why he was special. His spirit was whole and beautiful, but his body was not. There was something missing. My heart started to break as the reason he was special began to reveal itself.

When Conrad was around six months old, I became increasingly concerned with his lack of development There was something not quite right, I could feel it. I had been noticing small things for several months prior that worried me, in addition to some distinct preferences he had. For example: as he began to grow, I realized that his movements were quite jerky and stiff, his movements were not soft like babies usually are. If Matt or I tried to stand him on our laps while holding him steady he would keep his little legs bent up in front of him. I started to wonder if I had ever seen him straighten his legs. He was completely indifferent to sitting up or holding his own bottle or even trying to roll over on his own, and he absolutely hated being placed on his stomach. However, he loved to lie on his back watching the world around him. But he never kicked his arms or legs as I saw my other friends' babies do. At first I didn't even think about it as 'different' because he was so content. I did worry about him getting a flat head from lying on his back so often, that I would prop him up with pillows in a semi-sitting position, only to find him coyly smiling as he slowly inched his body back down into a horizontal position!

I remember going to the library with a friend and looking up books on cerebral palsy. (I have cousin with CP, and I thought that that was Conrad may have.) When she saw what I was doing she said, "Don't do that! You will just upset yourself." Well I was already upset! I knew something was wrong I just didn't know what.

As I watched other babies around his age or even younger the differences between them and Conrad became more apparent to me. For example he wasn't babbling or really making any sounds of significance at all except for laughing and crying. Other babies were babbling to themselves or to their mothers. He was silent. He didn't even make noises with his lips. It was as if he was stuck. I said to one of my friends that I wished he would just snap out of it, that he would wake up and begin to do the things that other children his age were doing. He had a very difficult time keeping his pacifier in his mouth, and as he wanted it all the time we actually resorted to tying a towel around his head to keep it in. My husband was certain that Conrad was a mellower child, unlike our older son who at the same age couldn't wait to sit up and roll over and crawl and hold his own bottle. I considered this but was not satisfied with him just being mellow.

During our son Ben's three-year well–baby check up (to which I had also brought Conrad), I expressed my concerns about Conrad's development to their pediatrician. As he was due for his one-year well-baby check, Dr. R. recommended that I come to the appointment with a list of my concerns written down so that we could go over them together.

I did as he asked and the next week as I sat watching, our pediatrician took Conrad in his large weathered hands. I could see the concern in his eyes. I blurted out before he could even say anything, "But he's not retarded right?"

He looked at me tenderly and said, "Well, he is retarded in that he has not reached some of the milestones other children his age have met already." I was floored but not entirely shocked. I didn't ask many questions, as I didn't know what to ask. I didn't know how to process the fact that he had just given weight to my concerns. He continued with his tests: gently testing his reflexes, monitoring his eye movements, and trying to get him to stand on his feet. He didn't say what he thought it could be. I am sure he didn't want to worry me with an educated speculation. He told me that he wanted to Conrad to see a pediatric neurologist, as his delays could be something cognitive. I left his office with the number for a pediatric neurologist, feeling if anything, numb.

My parents happened to be staying with us at the time, and when I came home I had to explain to them that there might be something wrong with their precious grandson. My mom was holding Conrad on her lap when I told her. She immediately started to cry and said, "Not Conrad, this sweet little boy." That was a really difficult conversation to have as I had to make a choice as to how I was going to handle all of it. I decided right there to be strong. Nothing was going to break me; I was going to be fine, no matter what. I had to keep telling myself this over and over. I was afraid that if I fell to pieces I might not be able to put myself back together. It seemed to work, because I was able to hold it together quite well.

I am not sure why, but I was terrified to let people know how hard it was for me to be faced with the fact that my son, our precious son, was different. I didn't want to be pitied or treated any differently. Mostly, I didn't want him to be treated any differently. I knew how some people treated people with disabilities; as less than human. I wanted our son, despite his differences to be loved and treated well by those around him.

I was suddenly thrown into this world of all consuming worry that our son had some kind of neurological disorder. I had no idea how to navigate my feelings. I had no one to talk to. I remember one day going to pick up my boys from a dear friends house, and as I stood in her kitchen, I was overcome with grief and I started to cry. She asked me what was wrong and I told her how worried I was for my little man. She did the perfect thing; she hugged me and let me cry. She didn't try to tell me that everything would be fine, or that I was worried for no reason she just let me cry. It was just what I needed.

A few days later my husband, Matt, and I took Conrad to see the pediatric neurologist. We were unimpressed, as he didn't seem particularly concerned, he just asked us a bunch of questions about Conrad's personality and what he could or couldn't do. This ambivalent behavior only led Matt to believe that Conrad was just a little bit slower than other children his age and would catch up. With an appointment in hand for Conrad to have a brain MRI, we left knowing nothing more than we had before, which only led to more questions.

After the MRI was performed I had to wait several days for the results. The waiting became unbearable so I called the neurologist's office to see if they had the results. The nurse informed me that the doctor had already left for the weekend but that she could give me the results. The results were normal. *Normal!* I was so excited, but now what? I asked the nurse to leave a message for the doctor to call me as I still had questions. He never did call me back.

A week later I received a call from my pediatrician, stating that he had spoken with Conrad's neurologist, and they both felt that he should be evaluated by the CDRC (Child Development and Rehabilitation Center), at Doernbecher Children's Hospital at OHSU (Oregon Health and Sciences University), in Portland Oregon.

I received a packet in the mail from the CDRC with pages of questions to fill out about what your child can do, can't do, your observations, and your concerns. I filled it out immediately and then waited for the day of the appointment to arrive.

We had to be at the hospital very early in the morning as we had been informed the appointment could take as long as four or five hours. We arrived on the seventh floor of Doernbecher and looked around. There were a lot of sick children and a lot of concerned parents and family members waiting. Conrad's name was called shortly after we sat down. I knew we were going to have answers that day, and I was anxious to get started. We started with a hearing and vision test, which he passed with flying colors all the while flirting with the technicians! We then moved on to the physical and occupational therapists. Seeing our son evaluated like that was tough as his ability to perform simple skills was very minimal or nonexistent. Conrad didn't seem to be bothered with the fact that these people were studying him, testing him, and judging him and his abilities. He just sat quietly and let them do their tests smiling all the time. Once the specialists had finished their testing we were told to go and get something to eat while they met to discuss their observations.

As we sat picking at our lunches with Conrad beside us in his umbrella stroller, seemingly oblivious to our concern, Matt and I discussed what these men and women would tell us about our precious son. Matt still held firm to the belief that Conrad was just a bit slower than other children his age and that he would catch up. I remember looking at this strong, tall, brown-eyed man that I loved dearly, and thinking it is going to be so very hard for him when they tell us that there is in fact something acute affecting our son's development. I felt guilty for not only believing, but also somehow knowing obvious to me. Why wasn't it obvious to him? I can only attribute this to the fact that Matt is an eternal optimist. It was excruciating being the only one knowing it would be bad news when he believed it would be good. We sat in our own thoughts until it was time to go back to the conference room where we would be told the news that would forever change our lives.

Finally it was time to meet with the specialists. We were ushered into a conference room where we sat down and waited for them to tell us what our son had. The doctor in charge of our case spoke for everyone. I have no recollection what she said to us, I just remember her being very kind and tender as she told us that they believed our son had Angelman syndrome. *Angelman syndrome? What is that?* I thought to myself. They began to explain it to us, but my head was in a fog. All I remember hearing was something about a small head and developmental delay and a blood test.

Before I knew it we were in a small room, holding our son down while his blood was drawn in order to determine for certain that he in fact did have Angelman syndrome. The nurse who took his blood told us it would be about two weeks to get the results.

I used the time between awaiting phone calls to research Angelman syndrome. It was difficult to find anything helpful. A woman at church approached me that Sunday with a thick envelope (she worked with children with special needs in the classroom and was curious about AS). The envelope contained a transcript written by a mother of an Angel at a conference on Angelman Syndrome. I began to read it the minute we came home from church. As I immersed myself in the pages, I became more and more alarmed. As I read the transcript I delved into a world that was full of enclosed beds, locks to keep angels out of bedrooms and bathrooms, duct tape on diapers, footed pajamas with the feet sewn on backwards to avoid children getting into the mess, no sleep, and even the locking of a child in a closet with bungee cords during hotel stays. I was horrified and scared to death. How could this be? I couldn't possibly have to lock my child in his bedroom at night or modify clothing in order to prevent him getting into his diaper and paint the walls with what was inside. The mother also mentioned the constant worry and stress of seizures, sleepless nights, and countless medications. The sheer amount of work these parents took on to keep their daughter safe, busy, and interactive was monumental. I was simply exhausted from just reading about their life. I was scared that might be my reality. How would I be able to do all that was needed of me? Where would I find the money to buy all of the modifiers that they said were essential in raising an angel? Where would I find the energy? Would I be able to rise to the challenge? Could I rise to the challenge?

I was completely overwhelmed by all the information that I just sat in my chair, numb, with shoulders slumped in submission. I don't know how long I sat there before I decided that that might not be the case with our son. How could I possibly know from reading one person's experiences that we would have the same experiences? As horrifying as this one woman's experience with her Angel daughter appeared to me, the overwhelming love that she felt for her daughter was evident throughout the manuscript. She did everything in her power to protect her and to make her life as safe and as stimulating as possible. I don't remember if my husband looked at or even read the transcript. He is not the type of man to worry and anticipate what he will do if this or if that happens; he tackles a problem when it presents itself. I decided to handle the information in much the same way: I determined I couldn't be afraid of a reality that may or may not be ours.

The greatest thing that happened to me during this time was I started to run. A few of my girlfriends were training for a 5k, and they asked me to join them. It was the perfect diversion for my mind. I was able to focus on something other than what I was going through with

Conrad. Running granted me strength. It also gave me uninterrupted time to think about nothing other than the next mile. It was a source of therapy and escape for me. Whenever I finished a run I felt like I could conquer anything that came my way. It also provided me with the strength to handle all of the appointments that were required to help Conrad become as strong and as self–reliant as he could be. I had a much better outlook towards the future with a disabled child.

In just under a week I received a phone call from the CDRC, saying that Conrad's blood test had come back positive for Angelman syndrome. Another appointment was set up to meet with the genetics team to discuss our son and his disability. We were advised to prepare a list of questions to bring to the appointment, as we may not remember all that we wanted to discuss once we were there. The night before the appointment I sat on our bed and discussed with Matt what we wanted to ask I kept that piece of paper with the questions I wrote down:

- Questions for the geneticist

- How independent? Walk? Talk? What are the expectations?

- Will he go to College?

- Will he get married? Have a job?

- Will he have kids? Will his kids have it?

- Life expectancy? Quality of life?

- How did he get it?

- Can our future kids get it?

- Group home?

While waiting in the small cream-colored room, sitting on painfully hard chairs, looking at meaningless shapes in strange colors stenciled around the perimeter of the room, I realized that I already knew the answers to most of the questions I had scribbled down the night before. Only one unwritten question now mattered to me the most: *Would Conrad know that we love him?* I don't know why I felt a professional could answer this. After such a negative diagnosis, perhaps I just felt I needed to hear an authoritative "yes!" I knew in my heart that Conrad would never go to college or get married and have children of his own. But surely he could know that he was loved! It was as if by knowing this all of the pain and worry would be manageable. Four people entered the room: an elderly female doctor who was the genetics team leader, two of her team members, and a genetics resident. With little introduction, the lead geneticist pointed to the spot on Conrad's DNA chart indicating a partially-deleted fifteenth chromosome. Our son, indisputably, had Angelman Syndrome.

I have no idea what happened next or exactly when I asked if my son would know that we love him. The geneticist paused, looked expressionless at Matt and me, and gave a safe and presumptive medical answer: "No."

Even today, I cannot find the words to describe how I felt at that moment. I could barely breathe. I was sweating and choking on the lump in my throat. I knew the doctor was continuing to talk, but I was drowning in deafening silence. Somehow I had gotten myself to the sink where I was trying to retrieve a paper towel to wipe my face and blow my nose. I remember asking for a minute to catch my breath as this unimpassioned woman droned on about DNA and chromosomes.

Finally, after tremendous effort I was able to collect myself. I didn't dare look at Matt, who was clearly struggling to retain his composure for both of us.

We were both offended by the clinical way the geneticist spoke of our son, as though he were not a real child. That was almost more upsetting to me than being told he wouldn't know we loved him. At that moment, I knew she was wrong. Conrad did know that we loved him, because he certainly loved us. He couldn't say it, and he still hasn't said it, but he shows us every day that he loves us, and we show him every day that we love him.

The following is a letter I wrote shortly after Conrad's diagnosis:

Dear Conrad,

On June 26, 2003, we found out that you have Angelman syndrome. This is a rare genetic disorder that is in effect a deletion of chromosome fifteen. We found out on a sunny day up at Doernbecher Children's hospital. It was a very difficult day for your dad and me. It was an even more difficult few months to follow as we struggled to comprehend and accept what was happening to our smallest boy. It never changed our love for you, just our perspective on how fragile life is, and yet how interesting and how blessed. The three of us (Dad, me, Ben), have all dealt with it differently. Ben prays all the time for you to be able to chase him. He is getting to know you and is always very sweet to you, except when you pull his hair. Dad has a huge soft spot for you and loves to spend time with you. I love your infectious giggle and don't know what I would do if I couldn't hear it everyday. We love you and your spirit and how you keep us close to God and to the Holy Ghost.

Love Mom, Dad, and Ben

Connie has not suffered from many of the characteristics often associated with Angelman syndrome, in particular, seizure disorder. He takes no medication, except Melatonin for sleep, and eats everything (except eggs), and an occasional item *not* found in any food group. He's swallowed a ring and a Chuck E. Cheese token, both of which required an emergency trip to the hospital. (My husband keeps both treasures as mementos.)

Two years ago, Conrad did have two febrile seizures, due to the onset of a virus. It was absolutely terrifying as I watched his face turn a dreadful shade of grey and his lips turn blue. I know that there are some children who suffer from seizures several times a day, and my heart goes out to those who are dealing with this agonizing element of Angelman syndrome. Not a day goes by when I do not thank the heavens that we do not have this challenge with Conrad or wonder why we were spared from this exhaustive trial.

For the first three years of Connie's life, he did not sleep. As a result, neither did I. There were days when it hurt to open my eyes, let alone move. I would stay up late with Connie, balancing him perfectly on my chest (as that was the only way he would drink a bottle), using one hand to hold the bottle and the other to play Free Cell or Solitaire on the computer. (For several years after I had constant pain on my chest where he had laid that made moving or getting dressed a painful exercise). I'd often bring him in to sleep beside Matt, who, to this day, seems to have a calming effect on Conrad. He was Connie's Melatonin long before we discovered it!

I recall one day being especially frustrated with Conrad while trying to make dinner. I was in the middle of cooking, I was worn-out, and I couldn't stop what I was doing to feed him when he wanted. So I grabbed his bottle, propped him up on the floor beside where I was cooking, and told him, "Conrad this is your bottle, this is how you hold it, I need to cook dinner, and you need to drink your bottle." And he did it! From then on he fed himself. I have since learned that when I need Conrad to learn a new skill or we are somewhere new, if I take the time to explain to him what is going on, he listens and will usually obey or calm down.

Conrad has acquired many nicknames over the years. Our favorite is *Connie*, the name we use most often. There's also *Frog*, *Corndog*, and *Slick*, which he earned after discovering an open jar of Vaseline. Then there's *Conradical*, (a family favorite) given to him by his namesake, Uncle Jefferson.

Since the day we found out about our son's diagnosis we have worked very hard to provide as normal a life for him as possible. He has three brothers who adore him and love to make him laugh by being goofy. All three boys have been vital in Conrad learning to do so many things such as: drinking from a straw, learning to use a fork, walking, swinging on a swing, wrestling, washing hands, going potty, and bringing one of us the remote when he wants to watch TV. Our son George said to me once, "Conrad is cool because he doesn't talk."

Before Conrad was independently mobile, my boys and I had been invited to play at an indoor play land at a fellow Angelman mom's church. As soon as we arrived, the twins, George and Wilson, were running around playing with all the ride-on toys they looked over to see where Conrad had gotten to when I saw him looking up at the back pockets of my mom's jeans. I could, imagine his internal dialogue, "Ah! Pockets! Now if I can just grab a hold of them I will be able to stand up." My mom about fell over when she felt someone touching her behind! She laughed hysterically as she realized Conrad only wanted to be up on his feet. I can't count the number of times I have almost dropped my drawers as Conrad has taken a hold of my back pockets in order to be upright!

One afternoon after I had just finished giving Conrad antibiotics for something, Ben asked me, "Mom when is Conrad's Angelman syndrome going to get better?" He didn't realize that AS was a permanent condition. His question surprised me as I realized how thoughtful and profound it was.

His question, so innocent in nature, pulled at my heartstrings. I paused for a few moments as I contemplated how to answer him in a way that he would understand. I told him that some people come to earth in imperfect bodies so that we might learn things we may not otherwise learn, such as patience, endurance and love. We discussed all the things that we had learned from Conrad so far. When I asked him what Conrad had taught him, he responded that he had learned that even though people may look or act different, they are just like us: they like to laugh and be played with. I also told him that his situation was only temporary, that while on this earth Conrad would have AS, but after he passed on he would be released from the binds of his disability and would be able to do all the things that he is unable to do now, like talk and run and jump on the trampoline. Ben listened intently, and when we were finished talking, he said, "Mom, I can't wait to hear Conrad's voice and play tag with him!"

Conrad is very motivated to keep up with his brothers, however, and we are pretty sure he will be running right along with them in no time.

Life with Conrad is not easy, and there are days when I feel that I can't do it anymore; the constant supervision, changing, dressing, feeding, sleepless nights, messes, and just the knowledge that I have a son with a disability is tough and sometimes heartbreaking. Sometimes I feel like I am missing out on life and the things I could be doing if I weren't keeping track of Conrad's every move. For instance during Ben's basketball games, Conrad would love to run out on the court and be with the other kids and hug them all. We would love to go camping as a family, but this is nearly impossible as Conrad will not sleep unless he is in an enclosed bed or heavily drugged. Even then I am not sure he would sleep. I would love to go hiking on a Saturday with the entire family, but physically Conrad is not there yet. The list goes on and on. I fight the urge to feel sorry for myself as I watch or hear of other families doing the activities I long to do with mine. It is very challenging.

We have had to adapt to the lifestyle we have and not distress over the life we don't have and may never have. We do however have respite care during the week and we receive one twenty-four-hour period per month where we are able to take our other three boys to do things that we are not able to do with Conrad—yet.

A few months after Conrad was diagnosed I was sitting at my mother-in-law's desk when a pamphlet from her dad's funeral caught my eye. I picked it up and started reading. It described the different stages of grief one goes through after losing a loved one. I recognized right then that I had been grieving for Conrad, for the life he was not going to live, the life we were not going to live. According to the pamphlet I was in the last stage of grief, which is acceptance. I had begun to accept the life I had been given. We were in a good place in our life; Conrad was going to therapy and to Early Intervention every week and was making progress. I was getting used to the fact that I had a son with a disability and a rare one at that. I had begun to thrive in my new life, and I felt blessed to know this boy and to learn from him.

It has not only been our immediate family that has been blessed to know Conrad. We have had many friends and acquaintances that have spoken to us in private or sent notes about how he has touched their lives.

Dear Sister Lyman,

I have never thanked you for the wonderful opportunity I had to work with your son in the nursery. He is a special gift from Heavenly Father and is a great example to me. I suppose the best way for me to convey this message is to give you a few examples of the love of Christ I witnessed through his actions.

Once, there were two girls in nursery who had a little disagreement between them and were separated into different corners. Conrad saw their sad and upset natures and promptly scooted over to one of the girls to provide comfort. He tenderly tried, but because of the nature of this girl, she said, "No Conrad, this is my corner." He seemed a bit confused, and yet, still concerned.

Another day, Conrad approached Kyler in a playful spirit and they proceeded to tickle and gently wrestle each other. As Kyler noticed me observing, he said, "Look, Conrad likes me, we are friends!" For the rest of the day, they continued to play together, huddling under the table and giggling.

After one week of noticing Conrad diligently watching us play *Ring Around the Rosie*, I decided that we would try to help him to be able to play, too. And so, the next week, I held him up, and with the other children holding his hands, we walked around in a circle. I was so excited for him when, the part of "We all fall down" came, he seemed to buckle his knees and fall with the other children.

As we gave the lessons, I loved to watch the joy in his eyes when he saw the pictures of Jesus and looked at them in great focus. Then look at the other children in observance.

Conrad is an especially great Spirit. He taught me that I wanted to work with children like him. To be able to see their eyes when they have learned something; physically, spiritually, and mentally, it is something special. You can just see the love of Christ emanating from him. Thank you for diligently working with him and teaching him Christ like virtues. He has certainly retained them and works to apply them.

Thank you again,
Kendra Titensor

One instance in particular I was fortunate to witness for myself. We were entertaining a business colleague and friend of Matt's in our home one evening. He had just lost his own dear grandson to Angelman syndrome a few months earlier. Tom had not had the opportunity to meet our children before this point but knew that our son shared his grandson's disability. Tom was sitting in our kitchen when Conrad walked into the room and saw Tom. Before I could introduce them, he grabbed this total stranger in a huge bear hug. Tom was overcome with emotion as he moved to the couch to revel in this sweet display of love from a child he had never met. Tears ran down all our cheeks as we watched our son comfort our friend. Afterwards Tom said that while Conrad was hugging him he felt as though Conrad knew he had just lost his grandson and was consoling him. It certainly looked that way to us.

Conrad has an ability to console those who are unwell or feeling down. Only a few months ago my own brother was going through a difficult time in his life and was spending the day with me. Conrad happened to be home sick that day from school. We decided to go out for a short walk. As we were walking, Conrad kept stopping my brother by grabbing his sweatshirt and pulling him closer and catching him in a hug. He continued to pull on his sweatshirt until he finally had to stop in order not to fall over from his constant tugging. Conrad caught him in a bear hug and, as he was holding him tight, my brother looked at me with tears in his eyes and said, "Wow, that is pretty sweet." My brother had to finally carry Conrad on his back or the two of them would have been stuck in a hug for the rest of the afternoon!

A few years ago, my mother-in-law, who is the CEO of Special Olympics Oregon, was presenting a Leadership Conference for the organization's key volunteers. At this annual event, she would provide a heartfelt update on her grandson, Conrad. For four years, her closing remarks were, "He's not walking yet, but we know he will someday!" It was a message met with knowing nods from an audience who had never met Conrad, but knew very well that special needs children write their own stories. Finally, like a graceful but gangly newborn giraffe, Conrad took his first steps—at four years of age. He had written the next chapter of his story. And he was immediately cast as the headliner of his grand-mother's next conference. That year's theme of "Old Hollywood" – including a red carpet – was the perfect setting for Conrad, the star performer.

As my mother-in-law jubilantly announced her grandson's great new accomplishment, Conrad clearly knew that he had a special role to play—in fact I could hardly constrain him. He broke free of my grasp and headed up the aisle, upright and walking on the red carpet to give his grandmother a hug and to take his place on stage. No movie star could ever have been more loved or enthusiastically cheered than my son on that day. Fully enjoying the applause and accolades, he continued to "work" the crowd, stopping to touch someone's hand or give a hug. He knew that these peo-ple were clapping for him: he could sense their joy in the fact that he was walking and he relished so fully that I actually thought he might take a bow. At one point, he reached out for a particular woman, promptly sitting on her lap and giving her a big "Angelman's hug." For a second I wasn't sure if I should think, "*Oh cute*", or, "*Sorry! Let me grab my son from your lap!*" but she enveloped him in a wonderful hug of her own and with tear-filled eyes told me that she knew how special these children are as she had a daughter with Down syndrome who had recently passed away. "I was feeling low today," she said. "Conrad knew I needed a hug".

It is at times like this that I realize Conrad is not just here as my son, he is here as a teacher and a healer. He is able to perceive the need in others to be loved in a way I have never known. I have been the blessed recipient of one of these special moments many times.

Often I have imagined what life would be like without a disabled child. Without Conrad, we could jump in the van and go on a hike as a family. With Conrad we have to leave a parent behind, or find an experienced caregiver. Without Conrad, we could go on an overnight trip where we all just crash in any hotel. With Conrad we have to convert a hotel room into a Conrad free–zone with an enclosed sleeping area, a TV with Cartoon Network running all night and an impossible silence by all family members during Conrad's sleep time.

I long for spontaneity. I long for the unachievable. I long for freedom. And the yearning that accompanies those feelings can be all consuming, knowing that there are certain things you will never experience with that particular child or with your family as a whole. I want to just up and go. I want to take all my boys on a camping trip. I want to erase the phrase, "We can't do that because of Conrad" from our family's lexicon.

But then I look at Conrad, really look at him, and I know that I would not want him any other way. Whenever I am feeling low or discouraged, I just have to look at Conrad and feel his great love for me and know that everything is going to be fine. I know that

Conrad is not going to accomplish all in his lifetime that we want for our children, like college, learning to drive, a first kiss (although he is showered with them daily), dating, marriage, children, and other of life's benchmarks. But when I contemplate his future, I see love, friendship, and the opportunity to touch the lives of many more people. As long as he has love and his family, all is right in his world.

In this life Conrad is an immeasurable gift. What seems a challenge is in fact an opportunity. What seems a sacrifice is in truth a blessing. I am as a mother -we are as a family—stronger in every way because Conrad chose to be a part of our lives.

My husband and Conrad have a very special bond that I am not privy to but love watching from afar. They are two peas in a pod. As soon as Conrad sees his dad, it is everything he can do not to turn himself inside out. Conrad loves to be as close to him as possible. Matt has often said that his ears are actually handles that Conrad uses for bringing him in closer to his face. Matt's favorite time of the day is when he gets to sit on the couch with Conrad and snuggle. They could sit in the same spot for hours, watching anything from golf to the history of the airplane. I often joke that the reason Conrad came to earth was so that he could sit on his dad's lap, snuggle, watch TV, and eat chocolate.

Conrad is loved by so many and has touched our lives in ways that I never imagined a child could. His brothers call him Connie and love to make him laugh by being goofy or making up crazy dances and songs. We are fortunate to live by several cousins who adore Conrad and play with him in their own way. It warms my heart to know that they love him and accept him no matter his abilities. For Connie's birthday his eight-year-old cousin Alex made him a PowerPoint presentation, because he knows how much he loves to watch TV.

One day while I had my six-year-old nephew, Isaac, over to play, I noticed Conrad sitting by the sliding glass door watching the kids play outside. I was disheartened that Conrad wasn't able to participate when I saw that Isaac was not outside playing with the other kids, he was sitting with his back to Conrad watching with him. He had chosen to stay and keep his cousin company. I wiped away the tears as I watched these two cousins share a moment quietly together.

For a long time I felt abandoned by some of my friends because of Conrad. I felt polarized as calls to join in playgroups stopped coming. I was now the woman with the *handicapped child* and no longer had anything in common with these other women I had considered my friends. I discovered that some people found his disability too difficult for them to be around. People didn't know what to say to me or how to act around me. Thank heavens I had the support of a dear husband and a handful of empathetic family and friends to buoy me up. I was lonely and confused to be shut out because of a diagnosis. But fear is a powerful thing. Thankfully I found the strength to move forward.

It was during this time that I discovered a new friend and confidant: Hope.

> For we are saved by hope: but hope that is seen is not hope: for what a man seeth, why doth he yet hope? But if we hope for that we see not, then do we with patience wait for it.
>
> Romans 8:24-25 (KJV)

Hope became a motivating force for me as I became determined not to let our son's diagnosis rule our life. I decided that this life we had been asked to live would be rich in love and hope and miracles. Conrad was going to be a vital addition to not only our family but also the world. Because of hope I was able to heal my wounded heart of the concern and sadness I had about my son's diagnosis. It was not going to define our family. Conrad was Conrad, not our son with Angelman syndrome, no more than Ben was our *normal* or *typical* child.

Because of hope I have a stronger belief in God and know that He is mindful of us and that He knows us and know our struggles. I also know that patience is one of the greatest and most powerful characteristics we as humans can posses.

I am truly thankful for the opportunity to have in our family a true treasure in Conrad. He has taught me the power of the human spirit—that by your own volition you can accomplish much, that love is healing, and that laughter really is the best medicine. I am also thankful for all that he has taught our three other boys about adversity, perseverance, love, and hope.

I have no idea what the future holds for Conrad or for our family. We have been asked several times what Conrad's mortality rate is and what our plans are for him as he nears adulthood. Children with AS generally have the same life expectancy as anyone, barring any illness or accident. No one can predict what the future will bring for us or for our children. We certainly didn't predict that we would have four boys, one with special needs, one singleton, and a set of twins!

One thing is for certain—if Matt and I are lucky enough, we will still be receiving hugs, walking hand in hand, snuggling on the couch watching TV, and making Conrad giggle for many years to come.

PART TWO:
YOUR STORIES

CONRAD LYMAN

I always find it interesting to see what insight others have into different situations. It was very touching to read about how my parents view, not only Conrad but our other boys as well.

OUR ANGEL GRANDSON

By Jean and Chuck Blumenauer
Grandparents to Conrad Lyman

Conrad was born March 30, 2002, to Pamela and Matthew Lyman, our daughter and son-in-law. He was a beautiful blue-eyed baby with a halo of golden blond hair. He was a happy baby who smiled and giggled most of the time. During that first year, though, it became apparent that Conrad wasn't reaching natural milestones like sitting up and attempting to crawl. This was a concern for his parents, and they decided to consult their family pediatrician to discuss these issues with him. Conrad underwent genetic testing administered by specialists, and they determined that he had Angelman syndrome, a rare genetic disorder. None of us had even heard of Angelman syndrome. In the days and weeks that followed, we came to learn more about this syndrome and its impact on Conrad and his family members. It was a life-changing experience for everyone.

However, we've come to know and understand that Conrad is much more than his diagnosis. He has shown us that life doesn't always go as planned. He is a happy, loving boy, and it is impossible to stay down when you are around him. He has a large, captivating grin and a bubbly personality.

People are naturally drawn to him, and he makes new friends wherever he goes.

Conrad loves listening to music, particularly the sweet, swinging sounds of Lawrence Welk and his orchestra. Only his great-grandmothers truly appreciate his love for Lawrence Welk's music! He is fascinated with water. Any container of water—a kitchen sink, a bathtub, or something as large as the ocean—serves as a source of never ending entertainment for him. He enjoys either bathing alone or with one or two of his brothers.

Benjamin, his older brother, who is seven years old, is exceptionally kind and patient toward Conrad; he treats him with a great deal of care and concern. His younger brothers, the twins George and Wilson, are among his greatest supporters. They give encouragement to Conrad and invite him to play with them.

Tender feelings were felt by Pamela the first time four-year-old Conrad boarded a bus, taking him to pre-school. Conrad found it difficult as well to leave the security of his home, however, he soon adapted to riding the bus and attending school. His teachers loved him, and George the bus driver became one of Conrad's greatest admirers.

Conrad achieved two important milestones in his life this year: he learned to walk, and he started kindergarten. He has made many friends with fellow students and teachers alike. He attends church every Sunday with his family where he has many admiring friends.

Conrad doesn't speak, at least not at the present time. Perhaps he may never tell us that he loves us. But, we've come to realize that there is more to expressing love to someone than saying it in words. There are the constant smiles and hugs, the expressions he gives, snuggles, the way his eyes light up when he sees us. His face speaks louder than any words can.

Conrad is growing up in a home filled with much love, laughter, and respect. His parents are committed to helping him realize his greatest potential, and they have the support and love of their large, extended family. Pamela and Matthew are ordinary parents doing an extraordinary job.

Conrad is the angel in our lives as he gives unconditional, all-forgiving love to everyone. Thank you, Conrad, for sharing your life with us.

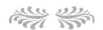

My oldest son, Ben, wrote this for a school assignment. I love that he is always thinking about finding a cure for his brother. Maybe, one day he will.

THE CURE

By Ben Lyman
Older Brother to Conrad

Once upon a time there were four brothers. All could speak and be in a regular class but one. The oldest brother's name was Richard. The brother that couldn't speak was named Jefferson. The third brother's name was Justin. The youngest brother's name was Todd. One day the brothers decided to go on a walk to talk about Jefferson. They went on a walk in the forest near their house.

As they were walking they saw a frog that had a test tube. The test tube was full of pink goo. The brothers asked, "What's in the tube?"

The frog said, "A cure."

The brothers asked, "What kind of cure?"

The frog said that it was a cure for jewel syndrome.

"Can we have some?" asked the brothers, "because our brother has jewel syndrome.

"Okay," said the frog, "but can I see him first?"

"Sure we live just up the hill. Come with us and you can see him."

When we got home we had to look all around the house until we found Jefferson sitting in the bath, trying to turn the water on. When the frog saw Jefferson, he poured the pink goo all over his head, and immediately the frog turned the bath on in order to help the goo go all over his body.

Jefferson started to talk. He said, "Thank you very much! I've always wanted to say, 'Just pass the chocolate,' and also, can I have a new bed and not a crib please!"

The brothers were so excited that they yelled, "One more minute of this craziness and we'll all need a diaper!" They called all their family members, even their grandparents in Utah and Canada! They said, "You will never believe what happened to Jefferson!"

The family members thought that something horrible had happened. But the boys said, "No, if you want to find out what happened, find out for yourselves. Come to our house this Friday at three p.m. And one more thing, bring lots of chocolate!

When they arrived at Jefferson's house, he answered the door and said, "Where's the chocolate?"

The grandparents said, "Jefferson is that you?"

Jefferson said, "Yes!"

The grandparents almost fainted, so they had a great party. After the party the grandparents said, "How did you get cured?"

Jefferson said, "My brothers met a frog in the forest with a test tube full of pink goo. They brought the frog home with them, and he poured the goo all over my head, and I was cured. This is the best day of my life. Thank you for curing me, Mr. Frog. I love you for that. Without you, I wouldn't be cured. Thank you very much! Thank you all for coming, and can I have some more chocolate?"

All of a sudden, there was a knock at the door. Everyone went to the door to see who it was. On the doorstep there was a chocolate fountain with a big bow on top and a card that said, 'To Jefferson, here is something you can enjoy with your whole family.'

Everyone smiled as Jefferson picked it up and took it in the kitchen and began to set it up. From now on there would be chocolate any time anyone ever wanted it.

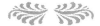

Alexander is my oldest nephew and one of the most fascinating people you will ever meet. He is always writing stories and making up games for his cousins so needless to say he was ecstatic to contribute a story to this book effort.

CONNIE'S BIG DAY

By Alexander Dale Lyman
Cousin to Conrad

Once upon a time Connie, Alex, Isaac, Jackson, Chase, Natalie, Jeff, Matt, Pam, George, Wilson, and Ben were playing in the backyard of Pammy's house. Then out of the bark chips came a magician who they had never met or known.

He said, "Connie come forth!" So Pam and Connie went to the magician.

"Connie, I hear you have some disabilities," said the magician.

Connie was scared. The magician's voice was thundering.

The magician thundered, "I have the power to take away your disabilities. You will become like one of the gang if you can complete this task. You have to jump off the deck to the grass three times. If you complete this task, you will become one of the gang for the rest of your life."

Connie jumped from the deck to the ground three times. He did it! Conrad raced to the magician, and the magician waved his magic wand. Connie flew up into the air, and a yellow light went out of him, and a green light went into him. He fell back to the ground. He stood up and exclaimed, "Yeah! I can talk!"

Auntie Pammy yelled, "Yeah!" And everyone else did too. Connie was now one of the gang!

The End.

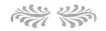

CONNIE

By Alexander Lyman
Cousin to Conrad

Conrad is very special. I love him. It's like having an extra special person who gets extra special care. I like to make PowerPoint for Connie, because I know he loves to watch things. That's how I show him I love him.

I hope Conrad learns how to read and write. It would make me feel really happy if Conrad could talk and tell me how he feels.

It helps me learn that some people can't do what others can do. If I see someone in a wheelchair, I'm not afraid of him or her I just want to help him or her. I will help them.

When Conrad got his play structure it made me feel special and good inside. I was happy that Connie got the play structure, because I could play with him on it. It was neat he had his own special swing. I like pushing him on it. It's nice to have something to play with that includes Connie. I love him.

Isaac is another one of my favorite nephews. He is always ready with a hug or a silly face for Conrad.

HUGS

By Isaac Lyman
Cousin to Conrad

Having Conrad as my cousin makes me happy. I like turning on shows for him and including him in our games. I like sitting next to him and saying, "Hi." My favorite thing about Conrad is that he gives hugs.

I hope Connie learns how to run so I can play tag with him. I want him to learn to play the Wii and the computer. I would like for him to play the piano too.

I've learned that some people can't walk, and when they try to walk, I help them by holding their hand. If they fall, I can help them get up. Heavenly Father loves everyone, even people with special needs.

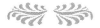

Natalie is the mother to two of my favorite nephews, Alexander and Isaac. She is more like a sister to me than a sister in law, and for that I am blessed. I love her sentiments towards all special souls. It is so true!

SPECIAL SOUL

By Natalie Lyman
Aunt to Conrad

There was a time that I did not feel comfortable around people with disabilities. It wasn't that I was embarrassed to be seen with them or that I thought they were less than me. Actually it was quite the opposite; I knew that people with disabilities were special souls sent to earth to teach others how to love unconditionally. I didn't know how to act around them. If I stared, would it hurt their feelings? If I looked away, would they long for my acknowledgment? As a result, I would end up sending an awkward smile their way, wishing I could be that person who was comfortable to hug freely or strike up a conversation. And then Connie came into my life; having Conrad as my nephew opened my eyes to many things. He taught me that people with disabilities want the same things everyone else wants—to be greeted when they walk in a room, to be hugged and snuggled with, to be told they are special, and to be loved. Every time I make an effort to connect with Connie, he shows his love ten fold. When I sit next to Conrad, he reaches out to hug me. When I greet him with a smile, he returns it with a laugh. When I hug him, he hugs me tighter. I no longer wonder how I should act around people with disabilities. Conrad taught me to treat them like I would every one else. I am blessed to be Conrad's aunt. I am grateful he is part of our family and look forward to all the other things he will teach me throughout our lives.

PRIYA MADISON ANAND

I had the pleasure of conversing with Nicholette first via email and then in person when we met at a conference on Angelman syndrome. Her submission was one of the first that I received so it holds a special place in my heart. I have read it over and over, sometimes laughing and crying at the same time!

LIFE IS WHAT HAPPENS TO YOU WHEN YOU ARE BUSY MAKING OTHER PLANS

By Nicholette Anand
Mother to Priya

"Life is what happens to you when you're busy making other plans..." The Beatles sang these lyrics, and my daughter Priya has certainly made me realize how true they are. Priya is six years old now and has taken us down a long and winding road that we would not have chosen, because it is so challenging, but she has nonetheless shown us many beautiful and interesting things along the way. She has definitely made us better people—more patient, stronger, more thoughtful, more clear about our values and priorities, more easygoing, and more compassionate. And all this under the duress of sleep deprivation—not bad!

Priya was born in March 2001; a beautiful baby girl with white skin, a pink rosebud mouth, tons of black hair, and beautiful blue/brown eyes. But, right from the start, I knew something wasn't right. Mostly, it was because of all her medical problems. She barely slept, cried all the time, had lots of gastro-intestinal distress, and finally, at two weeks old she developed a severe respiratory infection that put her in intensive care on a ventilator for three weeks. We were told she had a 50 percent chance of survival, and I remember literally getting on my knees and praying that she would be all right. Then doctors discovered she had two minor heart defects, a PDA and an ASD, which might require surgical correction later in life. I too had my own, non-medical doubts about Priya. When she was six weeks old I sat alone with her and looked into her big brown eyes; something in their expression made me think that something was lacking or out of synch and that she was in some way mentally handicapped. But of course I had no logical reason for this insight and certainly didn't express my doubts to anyone else. After all, what kind of mother thinks that kind of thing about her own child? At Priya's four-month checkup, the pediatrician commented that she wasn't yet holding up her head and seemed to have poor muscle tone. The doctor attributed this developmental delay to Priya's early illness, but I began to wonder. It seemed like each medical problem was a disparate piece of a larger picture that we hadn't yet managed to puzzle out. At six months we were referred to an ophthalmologist, because Priya had strabismus of her eyes. She also had lots of reflux and many breastfeeding problems that I was assured were *perfectly normal*, as was her erratic sleeping patterns. I went through life in a fog of exhaustion that made me wonder how other people seemed to function so well with their babies and didn't seem to find it as difficult and all-consuming as I did.

Despite this backdrop of medical and other concerns, we tried to resume normal life after Priya's arrival, and we focused on enjoying our pretty little baby who was so easygoing and smiley. But at eight months Priya still couldn't sit up, and we started being referred to specialist after specialist for test after test. Finally, in November, our physical medicine doctor told me that he didn't know what was wrong with Priya—why she was so uncoordinated and weak—but he assured me that something was very, very wrong. During this time I knew that we were going to get bad news, it was just a matter of what. My husband, Sanjeev, however, clung doggedly to optimism, saying he just knew she would be fine, and he found ways to poke holes in the logic of any concerning medical opinions we received. We each struggled to cope in our own way. For three months we went to countless appointments and began physiotherapy and occupational therapy. Every afternoon I would pack my little baby into the car for one appointment or another.

At some point during this period, the pediatrician decided to run a range of metabolic and genetic tests, "Just to rule out any problems and make sure we had nothing to worry about in that regard." She assured us it was routine and everything would probably come back negative. She advised us not to worry about it. So we didn't. Then on January 27, 2002, the phone rang at 8:30 a.m. and woke us up. I know it was 8:30, because that day stands out, crystal clear, in my memory. It was a Monday, and I answered the phone to find the pediatrician telling me it was her day off, but she would like to speak to us at her office rather than at the regular clinic. I asked what time, and she said, "Anytime, preferably right away."

I said, "Oh, we could come right now, as long as we're finished by about ten-thirty, because Sanj has to teach at the university at 11:00."

She said, "I think he'll want to cancel his class. He won't be in the mood to teach."

I was flabbergasted and silent.

She tried to reassure me by saying, "Don't worry, it's nothing terminal," but that didn't reassure me at all and only added to my confusion. How could it be so bad and yet not life threatening?

We flew into our clothes and arrived at the pediatrician's office within half an hour. As we sat side by side, she said that one of Priya's tests had come back positive for Angelman syndrome, had we ever heard of it? Dr. Davies was on the verge of continuing, fully confident that the answer was no. But I said, "Oh yes, I had recently read an article in a magazine about it. Children with Angelman syndrome can't walk until later in childhood if at all, and they are severely mentally retarded." At that point I realized what I was saying and started sobbing. Dr. Davies had tears in her eyes too, and we both just sat there as Sanj became increasingly worried and kept asking, "What? What is it? What's wrong? What's Angelman syndrome?"

We cried for days, and I walked around on the verge of tears for months. Passing songs on the radio, seeing young children in the mall, everything, and anything brought fresh realizations of our loss. Priya would never get married, never have children, never be an A student, never have a career, never share my love of reading, never run in the backyard and climb at the playground... The list went on and on, and although I forced myself to continue play dates with friends, seeing their children and hearing their discussion of them cut me like daggers to the heart. I grieved too for everything in our future that we were losing... thoughts of a child who grew into an independent adult, allowing us to travel and be carefree in retirement, hearing our daughter be able to say, "I love you," or tell me how her day was, or what she was thinking, all the *normal* experiences and rewards of parenting.

We went through all twelve stages of grief that people supposedly experience with the death of a loved one. And in a sense it was a death, the death of our idea of who our daughter was and would become. It was the death of many dreams, to which we were wedded more securely than we could have ever guessed. We went through denial (It couldn't be true; they should run the test a third time. Look how cute she is, how could anyone take away the future of such a little baby like this, they didn't know what they were talking about), then we decided she would be the exception (even if Priya did have Angelman syndrome, we would do so much for her and with her that she would surpass everyone's preconceptions and become smart and talk up a storm and she would walk and run like normal children). We didn't look up any information beyond the little we had been given, or contact any Angelman groups, for several months, because we were scared to learn any more potentially upsetting facts or predictions of the future. When we read of other parents' joy when their seven-year-old Angel started to walk, we were horrified and couldn't share that joy. We didn't want to be associated with any *group*, because we didn't want to belong there at all. We were fighting and resisting the diagnosis as much as we possibly could. My husband would walk to work crying and walk home crying every day for I don't know how many weeks. At first I was the strong one, because I was less shocked by the diagnosis and in some ways had been adjusting to the idea of a problem for a while. He had refused that idea until it was no longer debatable, so it seemed like more of a shock to Sanj. Over the years though, we have traded places many times, where he is strong, patient, and optimistic while I wallow in a pit of despair and sorrow. We take turns buoying one another up and are happy to discover on some occasions that we are *up* together.

Telling friends and family about Priya's diagnosis was very difficult, and we often didn't have the strength to do it. It would bring up such strong emotions for us; we would be unable to speak. Some people hurt our feelings in their reactions but most were sympathetic. What we needed from our friends and family required them to walk a fine line between sympathy and too much sympathy. Sometimes people looked at us with such pity and horror as if what we were telling them was so foreign and strange that they were completely unable to think of anything at all to say. This reaction just made us feel that our problems were somehow so rare and so strange that they were incomprehensible to others, and we were no longer part of normal society, no longer part of the life we so much still wanted to belong to. The friends who were most helpful were the ones who acknowledged that, although our situation was *big* and very upsetting, it wasn't weird or completely foreign. Our daughter's diagnosis and resulting disabilities were just an example of the big problems that confront people every day in normal life. People rightly pointed out that Priya was a wonderful girl, a fact that wasn't changed in the least by her diagnosis. This type of reaction made us feel reassured that AS was something we could get over, as other people got over deaths or illnesses or house fires, or whatever tragedies unfortunately strike us as human beings. Other friends were so upset on our behalf that they would cry and grieve with us. In one sense it was comforting to know that people cared so much about us and our precious little daughter. On the other hand it was emotionally draining having to comfort them when we felt so weak ourselves.

We thought we were strong at the time of diagnosis and were handling it all quite well. Looking back now I can see that we were a complete emotional mess for at least a year and really for two years as we traveled the long road to emotional acceptance of Priya's diagnosis. Gradually we learned to compare her only to herself, as the unique and special individual that she is. At most we perhaps compared her to other Angels, but less and less to other children her age. They slowly became another category completely removed from her. It would have been like comparing apples to oranges. It was no longer so painful to see what other kids at playschool were doing. We began to celebrate each of her little accomplishments and to really appreciate all she could do and all she was. We bragged about her learning to sit at twelve months, learning to sit herself up at eighteen months, learning to bum scoot at two-and-a-half, taking her first steps in a walker or holding our hands at about three, taking her first independent steps at three-and-a-half, crawling a few inches when she was six, and pedaling her bicycle independently for a few meters also at six. They were all big milestones for us.

We received excellent medical care at the Stollery Hospital in Edmonton, where we live, and at the Glenrose Rehabilitation Hospital. We also received many hours of ABA therapy from the Family Linkages Foundation of Alberta since the time Priya was two. But the one thing that was lacking, and its absence surprises and dismays me still, was psychological counseling. How could doctors provide such a devastating and life-changing diagnosis without providing emotional support for the parents? Shouldn't there be psychologists at the hospital specially trained to help families receiving such diagnoses for their children? There was lots of help for Priya: playgroups, physiotherapy, speech, OT, numerous medical specialists, AFOs, glasses, equipment, even child psychologists, but nothing for the parents. This oversight seems huge to me, and we talked to many other parents of toddlers with special needs, which were suffering and struggling just like us. We toyed numerous times (and still do), with the idea of seeking out private counseling, but what holds me back every time is feeling that a regular psychologist wouldn't really understand what we were going through. Sometimes it feels like no matter how much you explain and describe, people just don't really grasp what it is like; that's why talking to other parents in similar situations is so helpful. You don't have to explain in huge detail and tediously spell it all out for them to truly *get it* at a deep visceral level. Like old friends, even if you have just met them, there is so much they understand without having to be told.

Going to the 2004 conference of the Canadian Angelman syndrome Society was a big step forward for us. When we went in to hear the *welcome* speech, I was so scared I was shaking. I listened to the completely unremarkable speech with disproportionately tumbling emotions; at times I felt like laughing hysterically, and at times I blinked away the tears. I was so moved to see all the other Angels, big and small, and their families. During the week it became remarkably, and refreshingly, normal to see so many Angels. The anonymity of being one *normal* family among others was like a warm bath we reveled in. Nobody was whispering about us at the banquet, no one was being pitiful but kind toward Priya, no other kids were staring at her. If she made strange noises or waved her arms around, no one batted an eyelid. It was fantastic. The sense of community we gained from getting to know so many other families with preschool Angels, the inspiration of seeing so many parents of older Angels being so strong and positive, it all inspired us with new energy, new ideas, and new optimism. It was the final step we needed to get on with making the best of our situation. We left the conference armed with the ideas and strength to envision dreams of a future that didn't terrify or depress us.

And so, our day-to-day routines with Priya focused on learning the best information to help her and then trying to apply it. Our goal is to help her reach her full potential, whatever that may be. We make sure she gets exercise, works toward achieving her therapy goals, has lots of fun, and spends time with friends. But the daily routines are completely disrupted for one or two months of every year by bouts of illness. When Priya gets sick she is usually very sick, with grand mal seizures that can last up to an hour and require an ambulance. Here is an example of a late-night e-mail I sent to some friends in spring 2007, sharing what such an experience is like:

> Sooooo, it is now our fourth week of dealing with illness. Last week after I had poked a wee bit of fun at my husband for being a baby with his flu issues, I came down with it on Friday. Let's just say there was hurling, and I felt sorry for myself and had to crawl around at one point. Then all weekend Priya has been sick, still not better from the pneumonia she came down with three weeks ago. She has had a high fever and two attempts to have a seizure (we hit her with the big drugs before she got it firmly in her mind though). Then at 6:30 a.m. this morning Seraphina woke up and vomited all over the bed, ten minutes later on me, then on her fuzzy little *TV-watching chair* and finally all over the zillions of toys in the toy box—bulls eye!
>
> So after cleaning up puke and doing lots of laundry, I finally got Priya into the pediatri-

cian this afternoon, and after various tests we discovered she has a rare 1/100 complication from the pneumonia. Basically, she still has it in her left lung, there's now fluid in the lung, and something called a *cavitating lesion*—an area of the lung the virus has sealed off and is turning into Swiss cheese. So, after consultation with the infectious diseases specialist (no we're not contagious), she's now on a heavy-duty antibiotic and may be readmitted on Thursday for further IV antibiotics. And to make the situation that much better, my daytime help with Priya doesn't come when she's sick (just when I need them more than ever), because they're "only here to teach her." Oi vay. When does it end, people! I should just mention here that I have stocked up my pantry with a new bottle of sherry for Xmas, and I may be poking my head in there quite frequently in the near future... Better yet, there's always Priya's rectal Valium. Let me know if you'd like some, we're selling it cheap to friends instead of buying Xmas presents! (Kidding, really)

And that is the saga thus far.

Even in the midst of a crisis, we do try to laugh and see the funny side of *life with Priya*. Many of our more amusing stories involve, I am afraid to say, toilet humor that is not for the faint of heart. I am now utterly convinced that when I write my memoirs there will be a chapter called, *Illness* but also an even lengthier chapter entitled, *Adventures with Enemas*. For example... when we were first married, Sanj and I used to celebrate Valentine's Day by getting all dressed up and going out for an expensive dinner and perhaps to the theater. Oh, how times have changed! Two years ago we spent Valentine's in the waiting room of the hospital Emergency department with Priya crying her head off. We couldn't figure out what the problem was until her chronic constipation suddenly occurred to me. Sanj soon hurried in from the nearby pharmacy, and we disappeared into the ER's public bathroom to hoist Priya up onto the baby-changing table and administer a glycerin suppository. Well, before we could get her legs down, a jet of water shot straight out of her bum into my face and all down the front of my winter jacket. Sanj stared at me, mute with horror, and I think expected me to burst into tears or scream, or something drastic. These reactions occurred to me too as I stood there in shock, but then I realized that, really, it was pretty funny. What a ridiculous situation to be in on this particular day of all days, and what a contrast to our former *celebrations in style*. I couldn't help but to burst out laughing and chase Sanj around the tiny bathroom saying, "Happy Valentine's Day! Pucker up and give me a biiiig kiss!"

Our toilet humor has now expanded to include our youngest daughter, Seraphina, who has had a few of her own potty adventures thus far. For starters, she insists on cheering for me in public bathrooms just as she does for Priya at home, which is pretty embarrassing, and I have heard more than one person snort with concealed giggles in the next stall. I am tempted to say that Seraphina's arrival in our family was the *final* step in our healing. But really it is never final, so instead I will say it was one more *huge* step. She has helped me in particular to care less and less about Priya being different than other children. She has given us back so many of the dreams that we thought had been lost with Priya's diagnosis. Last week she responded, "I love you too," to me, and I was so excited! Seraphina runs around our house pretending to be a blue jay bird, keeping up a constant chatter, having numerous tea parties, reading books with rapt attention, and generally providing so many of the parenting experiences we were missing out on. I can't say enough about how funny or fun she is and how much we appreciate, and always will, every single step she can take and every word she speaks. It is a miracle I will never get used to, a gift for which I will never ever stop feeling gratitude. I often wonder if perhaps the diagnosis of Angelman syndrome is not quite so difficult or heart-wrenching for parents who already have a *normal* child. I imagine that it might not mean the huge and complete loss of hopes and dreams that it signifies for parents of only children.

Now, it doesn't really matter that we can't get these experiences from Priya. Priya is her own person, and I have far less need for her to be someone else. I can just appreciate all she is in her unique self. It is also really heartwarming to see how our two girls have developed a strong relationship and bond with very little intervention from either Sanj or me. Seraphina is

Priya's advocate and best friend, they love being around one another, and although they might fight over toys, they stick together in situations where they are afraid or unsure. Hearing twenty-four-month-old Seraphina tell Priya that "she a good boy!" was cute, but it was even more rewarding to see the big beaming smile with which Priya responded. She too has gained a lot by having a sibling.

When Seraphina was a baby and slept so much and was relatively easy to look after, it gave me new understanding of my time with Priya when she was a baby. It validated that I hadn't imagined how difficult it was; it wasn't my incompetence at all, those hurdles really and truly existed. In some indescribable way, Seraphina's movements, her biological rhythms, and her general development, all just resonated with me and synchronized with me in such a natural, easy way that Priya's never will. She made sense to me at some very basic level that Priya can't, because her central nervous system and her body are so different than those of a *typical* person.

Having another child wasn't all a bed of roses, though. The ease with which I could parent Seraphina raised in me resentment of how much more work it was to parent Priya. At one point I burst into tears and told my mom that I felt like Priya was a mistake and why couldn't Seraphina have been the eldest child? Maybe all the medical interventions that had saved Priya's newborn life were an unnatural meddling in the natural order. Maybe she wasn't meant to have survived, but should have just been a bright light that shone briefly

before being snuffed out as one of nature's cruel kind-
nesses. My mom sympathized but wisely reminded me,
"But then you wouldn't have known she had Angelman
syndrome. You would have thought you lost a perfectly
healthy daughter who would have had a perfectly normal life. And maybe that loss would be something that
you would never have got over either." We don't know
what the path less traveled would be like, and there
are no assurances that it would be happier or easier.
A friend was once at our house, and after watching
me take care of Priya, feeding her, etc., for a couple of
hours, she mused, "You are busy all the time looking
after her. I wonder what she did for you in a past life.
It must have been something really big." That thought
really struck me—that perhaps I really owe Priya a lot,
and everything I do for her is small compared to what
she might have done for me…

I try to remember these things when I'm having
a hard day and when my thoughts are running pell-
mell into each corner of my brain, like an animal in
a cage, searching for a way out of our situation. As I
tell my husband, almost every problem in this world
has a solution: you don't like your husband so you get
a divorce (no, not you honey!), you don't like your job
so you get a new one, you don't like your house so you
move, etc. But ongoing health issues, be it a stroke or
a diagnosis of Angelman syndrome, are not something
you can take charge of and simply or instantaneously
fix. You are stuck with them, period. There is no solution, no magic bullet. You can't will them away, and no
amount of hard work is going to make them disappear.

Angelman syndrome is something you have to work with and around, something you have to slowly incorporate into your vision of a happy life.

I used to think that a person's worth was somewhat determined by how smart they were, how self-aware they were, how kind they were, how interesting they were, what kind of job they had, how much money they made, which books they had read, and numerous other silly measures. Priya has made me learn that most of these things don't matter at all. To my surprise, my best friend in the world is a little girl whose tongue sticks out and who has no idea why Shakespeare is important or what NASA is. She has taught me that, in spite of all her limitations, her spirit is more precious and rare and valuable than many other people who don't face her challenges at all. In fact, she is a much better person than most people I know. She is kind and loving in an unconditional way that none of us more *complicated* beings can ever hope to achieve. Her emotions are pure in a way that I think God might perhaps be, shining forth with generosity and joy and unselfconsciousness. She is never happier than with other people, and she appreciates them for who they are, flaws and all. She remembers people for a long time and loves to cuddle and be a part of things, even if she can't directly join in. She is more than content to sit on the sidelines and watch others enjoy themselves. She is neither ambitious nor jealous nor selfish. She appreciates beauty and celebrates a special time when it is happening. Priya knows that chocolate birthday cake is a darn good thing and requires a second helping.

She is also perceptive. Priya knows when people aren't being genuine with her, and has made it clear that she doesn't want to spend time with them. Moreover, she has made me realize how caregivers of people with disabilities mustn't just talk *at* them or do things *to* them, they must recognize that each person has a soul and a personality and all the complex emotions people experience. It is important to follow their lead once in a while and to empower them with choices. It is *not* appropriate to be inanely, loudly, annoyingly cheerful and bossy all the time. Haven't we all absolutely loathed hospital nurses who are like that when we are feeing ill or weak or vulnerable? There must be times of laughter and cheerfulness, yes—and even guidance—but also times of quiet companionship, gentleness, empathy, and sensitivity to the idea that this is someone's life, and that they have an inner experience of their existence as real and as valid and as complex as any genius found in the membership of MENSA.

Although she can only say a few words—and those, infrequently—Priya has spoken loud and clear to me every day since her diagnosis. I marvel every day at how much she can communicate and how much she has made us grow without speaking at all.

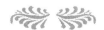

I love the unity that Evangeline expresses in her story that transcends language and cultural barriers. Angels are uniting forces.

ANGELS IN ASSISI: A GRANDMOTHER'S STORY

By Evangeline Rand
Grandmother to Priya Anand

The arrival of my first grandchild was a huge event in my life. She was a breath of beauty, an astonishing spirit to encounter. I fell in love with her profoundly. And yes, the announcement of her having Angelman syndrome was heartbreaking for all of us in the family. Indeed we have been set into trajectories of an education with enormous learning curves. At the time of her diagnoses I was also diagnosed with breast cancer. Life has certainly presented us with enormous opportunities to inspect it and ponder over it. I am left with a deep recognition of the staggering capacities of the human spirit—body and soul—to keep moving us into life's fullness and mystery. Don't for an instant get the idea that I am in any way diminishing the extent of the difficulties we have encountered!

I have to admit that I have never been that interested in *angels*—those we see in paintings from all the ages and different cultures, and which, now in vogue, adorn so many shops and advertisements. I had wondered about them. I had come to think that these previously portrayed angels were the result of someone trying to describe an experience that is really beyond description, and yet very real. Trying to elucidate the elusive seems to be part of our human task! Perhaps small stories have the same effect as *angels*, putting us in touch with fleeting truths, often ignored, that nevertheless can bring a certain quality of richness to grace our lives if we pause to engage with them.

I have just returned to Edmonton after facilitating a pilgrimage journey in Europe. I don't belong to any specific religious church. However, I do find it significant to travel to sites that have been revered as sacred, often for millennia, and which have been visited by crowds of pilgrims of different nations and persuasions, all of whom have left their homes and families, opening themselves fully to all the varied experiences of the journey; opening their hearts to receive and give *blessing*, or *Baraka*. Of course, such a journey can be experienced in just *traveling* into our garden or onto our balcony, or allowing our imaginations to take us on a pilgrimage.

The place of my special encounter with another Angel was in the small, medieval walled city of Assisi, Italy, the last site to be encountered in our pilgrimage. This site is ancient and predates the common era, but it is best known as the town where Saint Francis (b. 1182), and St. Clare (b. 1194), lived their love of all creatures, all people, and all of nature's fundamental forms, building a community of compassion, precious simplicity, and the courageous valuing of human truth. Of course, they weren't *saints* when they lived their lives! They were two young people facing the jagged interface of the overwhelming wealth of some citizens and the abject poverty of others. Their lives slowly evolved a healing story whose effect continues to ripple worldwide. Assisi is a place where you can feel the mysteries of life and love, the dignity of creation, in the very stones of the old houses, the curving networks of narrow streets—the soul of the town—and the cobbles you walk on.

I was coming down one of the winding, cobblestone alleys from the Saint Francis Basilica and found myself standing at a bend in the road, close to the open doorway of a small shop. Pilgrims have always loved to find small, treasured mementos of their journey, and I was no different.

As I approached the door, keeping my eyes lowered to help my feet pick their way through the crowd, I found myself noticing the wheels of a very special *stroller*. The thought that this would be a perfect fit for my granddaughter had hardly cascaded into awareness when I realized that the occupant of the stroller was a beautiful little girl, drawing me to her through her large clear eyes, her open and passionate smile, and her outstretched hand. A second later I realized I was face-to-face with another Angel. Thanks to the marvelous continuing education I have received, including the 2004 Canadian Angelman syndrome Society conference in my hometown of Edmonton, I have been able to perceive other aspects of the pattern of AS, such as certain arm and hand gestures, as well as larger body gestures of happiness and excitement.

I immediately stopped and took hold of the little outstretched hand, which caught the concerned mother's immediate attention. Of course, I knew why. She would not have expected a stranger to know how to relate to her daughter or to know how to avoid hair pulling, biting, and other possible sudden, erratic behavior. So I started to ask about her little girl. Someone from the crowd slipped forward to bridge the Italian–English language gap, "Yes…the little girl suffered from Angel syndrome…yes…this is a genetic problem…yes…it cannot be changed…yes…there are many difficulties, and yes, there is much love".

I quickly whipped out the photo I carry of my granddaughter Angel and her little sister, trying to tell of my deep appreciation of the situation. There were hugs and tears all around.

The little sibling of my Italian Angel was standing close by and was fully participatory, full of expectancy. She was a full participant in the moment and the mystery of our meeting. Our parting from the group resounded with, "Pace, pace"… "Peace, peace"…and the small crowd dispersed.

I was overwhelmed by the experience. Who would imagine that an Angel's grandmother from northwestern Canada would be drawn to another Angel on the other side of the world, at a bend in a very narrow, ancient street? Perhaps this strange type of synchronous happening is all part of developing a global consciousness.

After recovering my breath, I knew I wanted a *pilgrim's memento* of this special place and this unexpected and moving experience. After browsing in the shop for a few moments I found a very small *holy water* blessing vessel. I know I will probably forget to fill it with water on a regular basis, but I have since placed it directly opposite my front door so it can preside over all comings and goings.

I didn't know at the time that the extremely ancient symbol of the *Tau*, adopted and much loved by San Francesco (Saint Francis), was a complicated image that has accrued significance for thousands of years. It is the constant reminder to notice being alive and present in the moment, in the dark moment too. The *Tau* is there to remind us to keep breathing deeply, taking time to acknowledge that in and around us are the *angelic* energy patterns of life and love, taking time to admire in each other the triumph of the deep and enlivening spirit of true humanity. "Peace and all good!" was the old greeting in Assisi; it is still the greeting of today.

"Peace and all good," to all of us! Here's one grandmother who will be remembering it every day!

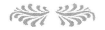

MY DEAR PRIYA

By Stacy Greening

A precious jewel

Who radiates with joy, acceptance and hope

Whose eyes sparkle with happiness and knowledge

With a spirit that embraces the challenges

And revels in the enchantment of life

You have shown us that life cannot put limits on joy

That there are no obstacles too large to overcome

And no limit to the love that you can give or receive

You find a purpose in life

And great hope for tomorrow

You have taught me that it is

Permissible to laugh and cry in the same breath

Allowable to entertain the excitement we feel

Especially when surrounded by loved ones

And that no day starts off badly enough that it cannot
be fixed

Priya, you are such a special person

And I am all the better for having met you

You have taught me more than any other

And I pray that someday I will be able

To teach you even half of what you have taught me.

CHARLENE BURBAGE

Devar's dedication to his sister's care and well being struck
me to the very core. I can only hope that my boys will be as
dedicated to Conrad once Matt and I are gone.

AN UNUSUAL LITTLE
GIRL AND HER FAMILY

By Devar Burbage

In nonmedical terms, Angelman syndrome is a bizarre, heartbreaking birth defect that presents families with extraordinary challenges, measured in physical and emotional dimensions. It is not life-threatening, but it presents families with serious lifelong problems to be faced.

A medical description of Angelman syndrome will be left to the professionals. Rather, this is the brief story of one family's long-term struggles to cope with the condition of a family member. It is a true story written with the hope that it will be helpful to others in similar circumstances.

There is no miracle cure at the end of this story. Instead, it is an account of a loving family dealing with the difficult realities of Angelman and somehow getting on with their lives while coping as best they could.

By the time Charlene was two years old, in 1948, it was apparent that something was wrong. While an apparently happy child, she had no speech other than squeals and gestures, and she was just then walking with difficulty and an awkward gait. The local doctors could shed little light on her condition, mostly suggesting that maybe she was just "a little slow in developing."

By age three, Charlene was no better, and it was evident something was seriously wrong. Her parents began making long trips to distant children's medical centers in search of treatment that would somehow cure their only daughter of this strange lack of normal development. The family was of modest means, and these trips were expensive and time-consuming. Nevertheless, the parents would let nothing deter them in their search for answers.

The answers were difficult to find. It took three years for them to locate doctors who seemed to understand enough of what they were seeing in Charlene to render opinions that seemed correct. The verdicts of several nationally known medical specialists began to converge. The consensus, in 1951, was that Charlene was profoundly mentally retarded, and would remain so for the rest of her life. Charlene's older brother, by five years, remembers the tears that were shed by Mom and Dad on the occasions when they were finally confronted by these difficult medical opinions.

By the time Charlene was six years old, she was a terror around the house. Nothing could be left out and within her grasp. She seemed to take fiendish delight in grabbing and dashing anything breakable. Her energy was boundless, and she rarely slowed down during the day. The simple, two-bedroom house was too small, and Dad decided he must add a room to make life more bearable for the family. The new room became that of Charlene's older brother, with a lock on the door on both sides. Brother learned to lock the door when coming or going to protect his model planes, school papers, scout projects, and anything else he valued that was breakable or could be defaced.

Charlene always seemed happy. She always had a smile. But she could handle few of the activities of daily living; she stuffed food in her mouth to overflowing, she could not dress herself, or bathe, or be left alone for more than five minutes. She still spoke only four words that could roughly be recognized as, *Mama*, *Daddy*, *cake*, and *candy*. She could no longer play unsupervised in the presence of other children without frightening them by grabbing toys and pushing, shoving, or hitting unexpectedly.

Behavior specialists suggested that intense, residential schooling at a special school might help Charlene. And where was such a school? The closest, and best for Charlene's needs, appeared to be the private Bancroft School in Haddonfield, NJ. This was 700 miles from Charlene's home in South Carolina, and these were the days before Interstate Highways. It would also be expensive for this moderate-income family.

Mom and Dad decided they had to do this, so they scraped together the initial money and decided that they would give it a try for as long as the money held out.

It was a long drive from South Carolina, consuming two full days, especially knowing what lay at the other end. Fortunately, Bancroft School was everything they hoped it would be: a very loving place with expert staff and happy residents. Nevertheless, it was difficult to drive away without their happy little six-year-old, Charlene, after only brief, several hour visits to Bancroft. They also knew that they could visit only rarely due to the distance. Air tickets would not be affordable, in view of the steep tuition. More tears.

Bancroft School was good for Charlene. The family had been told that placing the child in a daily routine that rarely varied was comforting to the mentally retarded. It was apparently true. She developed a bit more self-control and learned to submit to the authority of caregivers with less reluctance. The visits by the family (two days, one way, by car), every six months or so, revealed a happy child that was thrilled to see them, but had no problem saying good-bye and returning to her new playmates and caregivers. Thank goodness for small miracles!

After two years, Charlene's progress at Bancroft slowed to an imperceptible level. At first things had looked hopeful, with small steps in the right direction. But after two years the gains ceased, and the expense was a serious drain on the family. So Charlene came home to South Carolina at age eight.

Back home, Charlene quickly lapsed into her old patterns of behavior. The family had not the discipline and training of the school staff. Charlene resumed stuffing food in her mouth, grabbing things and dashing them, pushing and shoving and running around constantly. Only now she was bigger and stronger and thus more difficult to restrain physically. She was diminutive in stature, but strong otherwise and stubborn when she did not want to cooperate.

In those days there were no medications to help with aggressive behavior.

To help her awkwardness, dance class was tried. Charlene loved it, even learning one or two steps. Because of her unpredictable behavior, it was difficult for the teacher and other students, so Charlene withdrew after six months or so.

It was apparent that Charlene needed one-on-one care at all times. Loving, patient, private teachers tried to help her, but they really had no clue how to reach this child. No classes were equipped for that. Public schools were not required to provide for Charlene back then. Mom filled the one-on-one role at all times. It was an extreme burden, virtually twenty-four hours a day, except when Charlene was asleep for six to seven hours per night. An understanding, long-time sitter was able to provide some respite for Mom a couple of times a week for several hours each time.

It became increasingly difficult for the family to take Charlene out into the public arena. When she was a small child, a trip to a restaurant was no problem. But as a large child with behavior problems, Charlene was a serious challenge in a restaurant. She was quick and took delight in grabbing food off another table as she walked by, immediately stuffing it into her mouth. It was embarrassing, but funny, to see the expression on another child's face as Charlene snatched a muffin from his or her plate and ate it before anyone could move to stop her.

Charlene's Mom and Dad became active in Parents' Clubs, the Association for Retarded Children, Sheltered Workshops, and other civic initiatives that sought to push the government into providing better schooling and care for these mentally retarded kids of all levels. In concert, they were ultimately very successful in accomplishing their objectives, but it took many years.

Meanwhile, Charlene reached age nine, then age ten. She was still growing and becoming more and more difficult to handle. Medicines were primitive at that time in helping control her hyperactivity. Car trips were not too bad, so long as Charlene had her magazines to examine. Cookouts at the state park were a favorite of the family. Charlene could run around with nothing within reach that could be damaged.

By the time Charlene was eleven, it was becoming apparent that the family could continue to care for Charlene only with great difficulty. Attempts to provide Charlene with playmates mostly failed due to her behavior problems. She could not be left overnight with anyone other than her parents. Mom and Dad's network of parents with similar children was rather extensive by this time. They were the source of some social interaction for Charlene as they got their kids together for playtime each week.

Many of the other parents they met were facing and making the decision to place their child in residential care facilities. One close friend who was well off financially explained to them that he did not believe building a *gilded cage* for his daughter was the best thing for her. He wanted her to have social interaction with peers as well was being well cared for.

Mom and Dad had had a positive experience with residential care. Charlene had spent two successful years at Bancroft School and had been happy there. However, Bancroft was not an option due to the cost. They began to look around for other options.

In South Carolina there was an institution named Whitten Village, a state residential facility for mentally retarded and otherwise seriously handicapped people. It was named after the founder of the facility, Dr. B. O. Whitten. Dr. Whitten was still the director of the center and a master at squeezing money out of the state legislature for *his kids*. He had been hired as a young medical doctor many years before to run the fledgling facility and had made it his life's work. Thorough investigation and consultations with other parents of residents it was confirmed that it was a very well run facility. And it was only thirty-five miles away! And so, in September of 1957, at age eleven-and-a half, Charlene became a resident of Whitten Village.

Mom and Dad visited Charlene every two weeks. It was a family occasion in the early years, with older brother going along to help entertain Charlene. She always greeted them with shrieks of glee and ran to grab them around the neck. "We gotta go take Charlene for a ride," became a regular family ritual on weekends.

The routine at Whitten Center did not vary a lot over the years. She lived with other ladies of similar skill levels in a separate, small residential unit on a large, grassy campus under hundred-year-old oak trees. Her unit had several staff in constant attendance to the fifteen or so female residents of the unit.

Improvements in medications occurred over the years and were adopted at Whitten Center when appropriate. Charlene's behavior was definitely helped by the medications, designed to keep her calmed down to more normal levels.

Whitten Center provided numerous daily, weekly, and monthly recreational activities for the residents. Birthday parties, bus rides, meals at local restaurants, on-campus performances and festivals, Special Olympics, Sunday Church services, etc., filled their calendar.

Whitten Center had a very active Parents' Club. Dad and Mom pitched in to help in any way they could. Dad served as president several times. They raised the money to build a family center for family visits. The club eventually outfitted two apartments on campus where families could stay at no charge for overnight visits. The club was also very active in helping sponsor various seasonal activities such as Halloween parties, Christmas parties, Special Olympics, etc., year-round for all the kids at Whitten Center.

Whitten Center itself has gone through dramatic changes in the years of Charlene's residency. Doctor Whitten retired as director to great kudos for his years of service. Whitten Village's name was changed to Whitten Center. In the 1960s and 1970s the facility ran as high as 2300 residents. The advent of community-based residential centers dramatically reversed this growth, so that today it has only about 300 residents.

During their early retirement years, Mom and Dad spent the winter months in Florida, approximately 700 miles from Charlene. This stretched out the family visits, but they would usually make at least one trip home so that Charlene would not go more than six weeks without a family visit. Brother would often fill in for them when they were absent and at other times during the year.

On major holidays Charlene would come home for an overnight visit. In the early years these were multinight stays, especially at Thanksgiving, Christmas, Easter, Memorial Day, etc. Charlene loved opening gifts! What fun. She seemed not to care much what was inside. Easter egg hunts were also fun.

As Mom and Dad grew older, the overnight visits shortened to one night. They simply could not handle Charlene's hyperactivity and misbehavior for more than twenty-four hours.

The arrival of Charlene's two nephews on the scene added more family to the visits. Charlene loved to play with them on the visits as they ran around being young boys and treating Charlene as another playmate. They understood at an early age that Charlene was somehow arrested in childhood.

As age began to take more of a toll on Mom and Dad, their attention to their daughter became more and more difficult. Mom began to show signs of Alzheimer's, and Dad had several episodes with heart disease and stroke. Eventually Charlene's overnight visits home had to stop.

Finally, in their mid-eighties, a bad car accident forced Dad and Mom to give up driving. This was more of a shock than normal, since it seemed the end to the visits to see Charlene! But that was overcome by arranging for a driver to take them for their regular visits and to take Charlene for a ride. Mom's Alzheimer's was now in midcourse, and she understood less and less of what was going on around her. Nevertheless, she still made the trips to see Charlene, one of her deeply embedded memories that refused to go away.

Eventually, Daddy died. He made it to age ninety, largely on the determination to see to the care for his beloved Charlene for as long as possible. Mama continued to go with a driver to see Charlene every three weeks or so. Eighteen months after Daddy, Mama died suddenly at age eighty-six.

So now it's only me, (Charlene's brother), and my family, left. Unfortunately, I live 500 miles away from Charlene. I fly to see her as often as I can, about four or five times per year. I've also continued with the familiar driver, now with a nurse friend, going for a visit and a drive every few weeks. I think Charlene now considers them as surrogate *Mama and Daddy*, but who's to know what's in her mind?

Thirty days after the death of Mom, I got a call from a genetic testing clinic in South Carolina. It seems that they had done testing on Charlene for a few years at the request of Whitten Center and had found nothing… until the most recent time. This time they hit the right combination of tests and discovered that Charlene suffers from Angelman syndrome!

And so, at Charlene's age of fifty-five, and just after Mom and Dad had both died, this great mystery of what was wrong with Charlene began to unravel! The revelation came to me like a bolt of lightning. All those years of not knowing, and expecting to never know, suddenly at an end! Her condition has a name! Of course we don't know the root cause of Angelman, but even the knowledge that Charlene is a part of a population of similar sufferers is a breakthrough for me. I fired off e-mails in all directions to tell all our friends and family that now we know!

Charlene had been considered for Community-based placement on several occasions. She had even made visits to at least two of them. Her reactions to them were negative, and her behavior problems seemed to make it unlikely she would succeed at a small unit in a community.

But then another opportunity arose, Charlene had a positive reaction to the residence, and I decided to give it a try. That was in 2001, and it has been a big success.

Charlene is very happy in the community residence with seven other ladies and a staff of three to five at all times. A nurse is on duty one shift per day. She attends a Sheltered Workshop on weekdays where she receives training and social opportunities. Actual work has not proven possible in her case.

Many activities are planned and executed by the residence staff, some times together with other residences.

One unusual activity is weekly Sunday school at a local church that has adopted the residents and provides a special facility for them.

When I visit Charlene every few months, she is delighted to see me, with lots of hugs and kisses. After my visit, she has no problem going back home. I always spend additional time in the residence talking with the staff, letting them know of my keen interest in her welfare.

After ten years, her *driver* still takes her for a ride every couple of weeks, at my expense, and acts as a pair of independent eyes for me as to her apparent condition. He clearly sees it as his responsibility to help look after Charlene, even though he is paid. His monthly bill always has a handwritten note on her condition, for which I am truly grateful.

So that brings the story up to the present time! My sister is age sixty-one at this writing and a happy person in a settled, loving arrangement under the care and funding of the state of South Carolina.

Looking back fifty years, I believe my parents made a wise decision in the best interests of all the family, especially for Charlene, when they arranged for her to move to a residential facility at the age of eleven. I can attest to the fact from firsthand knowledge that Charlene considers her caregivers and peer residents as her family on a day-to-day basis. Charlene is happy in that environment. I know from frequent inspection over many years that she is well cared for. I also know that, even if she outlives me, her brother, she will continue to be well cared for by the never-ending stream of conscientious caregivers that make up her staff.

I'll end this story by saluting the wisdom and strength of Mom and Dad who made this tough decision fifty years ago, doing what they believed was in the best interest of their little angel. Time has proven their decision to be the right one.

KYLE TETREAUX

When I met Jennifer's parents and her brother Kyle they gushed about how lovely she is and how much Kyle loves her and her husband. I haven't met her yet, but both her parents and Kyle are lovely so I already know she is! I know you will love this story and get a laugh.

BURNED PLASTIC AND THE SIGHT OF FIREMEN

By Jennifer Moffat
Sister to Kyle Tetreaux

Kyle was eight years old when he was diagnosed. Up until that point we just said he was "mentally and physically handicapped." I was young enough that I don't think it occurred to me that it was strange that we didn't know what was *wrong* with him. My parents have told me stories about the things doctors said to them when they were trying to get Kyle diagnosed. Doctors who didn't know better called his AS other names. Some doctors who had no business being doctors accused my parents of malnourishing him or otherwise blamed Kyle's disabilities on them. Some doctors told my parents to put Kyle in a home and forget about him. One said he would never be able to "stack blocks," and he just wasn't worth it. I start tearing up just thinking about the things those people said. My brother, and the way my parents raised us, made me into the person I am today. I think our family is stronger, more compassionate, and more loving because of Kyle.

When I was younger I would sometimes feel a little bit embarrassed when strangers in the grocery store would stare at Kyle, but as I got older I just stared back.

Growing up with Kyle was at times frustrating, but really it was over little things, like him getting into my room (eventually I got a lock for it), or smashing my leftover birthday cake. I never felt like my parents favored him or put more energy into Kyle's care. My mom was never too busy to make me a costume for school. My parents never missed a volleyball game. I wouldn't change a thing about my family.

I love Kyle so much that if I even think about what it would be like to not have him in my life, I start to cry. What's so great about Kyle is that he doesn't have a mean bone in his body. He can't hate people. Anyone who will smile at him is his new best friend. He has this ability to draw people in and connect with strangers. He adores my husband and drew him right into the family. My scariest experience was probably the time he set a hotel room on fire. My dad and I actually weren't there, but when we arrived back my mom was outside holding Kyle with the fire department milling around. She had been packing our suitcases, and in a matter of moments Kyle knocked the ghetto blaster onto the stove and turned the stove on. My mom reacted quickly and there was no major damage, but the smell of burned plastic and the sight of the firemen were scary for me. (The whole thing was probably scarier for my mom!) There are so many *Kyle Stories* like that that I could go on and on. (Like the time he pulled a bungee cord through his cheek, or the time he poured water down the back of the television, or the time(s) he flooded the sink, etc.)

A hard moment for our family was when Kyle finished grade twelve. There was some debate over having him attend the graduation ceremony. My mom wanted him to be able to walk across the stage, but he was never a steady walker and seemed to get shakier as he got older. My mom went to the rehearsal ceremony and cried the entire time. She saw this gym full of students who were moving on with their lives, going off to college, starting a career, and Kyle wasn't going to have any of that. She felt like something was ending rather than beginning. I think it was also hard on my parents, because they reached the age where their kids should have all moved out. But they still don't have that freedom to just take off, whether it's to the grocery store or Mexico. We have been very fortunate in that we have fantastic people who do respite care for Kyle, but it's still never a spur-of-the-moment thing. Kyle still amazes us sometimes. He definitely understands a lot more than he can communicate back to us. He has only five words he uses (*mah-mah* for "mom" or "more", *pah-pah* for "dad", *buh-buh* for me, *ah-mah* for "grandma") and even those are iffy, but he can follow instructions like, "Close the door," "Give me your foot," "Go get in the car," and so on.

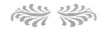

Kyle was the first Angel that Matt and I had ever met. I remember Dennis answering the door to their home and saying to Conrad, "I know that smile!" I steeled myself from getting emotional in front of them: but seeing Kyle for the first time was very difficult. He was in the backyard kneeling over a plastic tub of bubble filled water. I could not believe how similar he and Conrad looked. After I swallowed my emotions I said hello and sat down and we started visiting. It took him awhile to warm up to us. As soon as Conrad saw that there was water to play with he was right in there beside Kyle vying for a spot. Kyle wasn't too sure about this new guy getting in his space and let him know by trying to push him aside, but Conrad persisted. Dennis and Theresa were lovely to us: answering all our questions and not sugar coating their life with Kyle, but giving us hope, despite the difficult times. It was so nice to visit with them and see how much they adored him and how much he adored them. I will always hold that visit in a special place in my heart.

PEEK – A – BOO!

By Theresa Tetreaux
Mother to Kyle

We have a lot of Kyle stories and can't possibly tell them all! When Kyle was three, there was a World Expo in Vancouver, British Columbia. Kyle was in a stroller, and we were walking around, looking at exhibits. While in a line-up, Kyle reached out and grabbed someone's plastic bag and pulled a smallish gentleman right off his feet. The man cried out, sounding upset, but took one look at Kyle's smiling face and started to laugh. That same day, we were packed onto a boat on the fairgrounds. The woman standing beside us was wearing a flowing floral print skirt. Guess who started to play peek-a-boo with her skirt and ended up with his head under her skirt? The woman shrieked, grabbed her skirt, and yelled, "What on earth?" Guess who smiled back at her and batted his brilliant blue eyes? You guessed it—she melted on the spot, bent over, and gave him a kiss!

Dennis was speaking about IEPs at the AS conference in Colorado Springs in 1995. Den had a huge crowd at his final presentation, and as he was winding up, Kyle and I were walking by the room where he was speaking. Kyle heard Dad's voice, and right on cue, he dragged me into the room, let go of my hand, and walked up the aisle to give Dennis a hug, huge smile the whole time!

Our extended family has always had a really special relationship with Kyle. Jenn has grown into an incredible woman, and I think being Kyle's big sister has had a lot to do with it. On occasion when she has been asked what it is like to have a brother with special needs, she's replied, "Normal! I don't know life without him!"

We knew from an early age that Kyle was not typical. We spent a lot of time traveling to doctors and hospitals to get a diagnosis. Throughout that time our family and close friends were incredibly supportive letting us stay with them, babysitting Jenn when we had appointments, babysitting Kyle when we needed to spend time with Jenn or just with ourselves. Kyle's grandmothers both had heart-to-heart relationships with him. Finally getting the diagnosis didn't change anything, except that we had a *name* for what he had inherited, and we gained lots of new friends—the ever growing number of angel families.

What is their involvement today? It hasn't really changed. Kyle still travels with us to visit them, and he of course loves to spend time with grandparents, aunts, uncles, and cousins. Kyle's needs as an adult are a little different. His caregivers need to be physically strong and comfortable with changing him, so we don't leave him with family to be cared for. We have trained caregivers for that.

Kyle has made us value our family, friendships, health, and time. We like to think that we know what is important in life, and we take the time to enjoy every day.

We share the tough days with each other and add them to our growing book of Kyle stories. No matter how stubborn or challenging or sick or just difficult Kyle is being, there is always that smile! He loves us unconditionally, and we just have to remember that. We also make good use of our respite days!

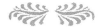

I WAS TALKING
TO SOMEONE

By Dennis Tetreaux
Father to Kyle
(Written by Dennis for Kyle
on his sister Jennifer's wedding day)

I was talking to someone…

I was talking to someone,

Who listened when I talked,

And asked about what I had to say.

I was talking to someone,

Who shared how she was feeling,

And wondered how I felt.

I was talking to someone,

And always looked on the brighter side of life.

I was talking to someone

Who thought about things

That were important to her,

And was interested in my thoughts.

I was talking to someone,

Who smiled as she told me a story,

And whose laugh lights up the space around her.

I was talking to someone,

Whose smile made me want to smile,

And whose twinkle in her eye,

Made me feel that everything was okay.

I was talking to someone

Who has lots of friends

But yet, made time for me.

I was talking to my big sister, Jenn.

With Love and Appreciation, Kyle

SARAH PATRICIA HERGOTT

I can relate to Leanne's feelings of hopelessness over the diagnosis of her daughter, becoming depressed and then slowly climbing out of the darkness and finding light in serving your child and family.

OUR PERSONAL ANGEL

By Leanne Hergott
Mother to Sarah

My daughter's name is Sarah Patricia Hergott. She was finally diagnosed at four-and-a-half years of age after many incorrect diagnoses. We naively hoped that she would grow out of her condition.

Sarah finally received a chromosome blood test after changing our pediatrician. Our old one moved away, and we had a brand new graduate from McMaster that started Sarah from scratch. The test was conclusive. We had a phone call three days before Christmas, 2001, and Sarah was diagnosed with Angelman syndrome. We were caught off guard and had no idea what Angelman syndrome was and its consequences. Thank God for the Internet. But after reading about it on the Internet we were very heart broken. Realizing that our daughter would never be able to speak to us and would be mentally and physically disabled her whole life was devastating. The good part of that time was that we were able to be with our entire family for Christmas and could tell them all at the same time. There were plenty of tears, and I believe that I was completely numb. It didn't hit me until after Christmas.

My reaction was later, when I became extremely depressed, angry, without hope, lost over thirty pounds, and constantly felt sick.

I finally sought the help of my family physician after hiding in a corner of my bedroom crying uncontrollably. I called my sister (from that corner!), and told her to take me to the crisis centre. She took me there and that's when my healing started to take place. I was not admitted to the hospital, but I did receive counseling and was put on antidepressants and sedatives. (Which I continue to use to this day!)

I had started to avoid my friends, my many friends, that I had for life, because I was so jealous and resentful that they had *normal* children. I became very antisocial and would have anxiety attacks if I ever had to take Sarah out. She would cry, scream, and vomit uncontrollably. She was very sensitive to anything outside of her comfort zone.

My husband on the other hand, dealt differently. He was very sad and withdrawn. He became angry but was angrier with me because of my behavior. He worked as many hours as possible and tried to stay busy and to stay away during bad times with Sarah.

I would have to say that I have had more than a complete recovery from my mental breakdown. Some kind of strength came to me and all of a sudden I saw my daughter in a different light, and I was able handle and embrace this life that I was destined to live. Once I became better, my family unit became better. I accepted that Sarah was special, and I made her into my *career*. I still worked at home in our family business, but Sarah and my husband, Paul, came first.

Sarah grew in so many ways. She had started walking at the age of three, but her general physical abilities are delayed but are improving at a slow rate. Sarah started sleeping with me as a solution to her terrible sleeping disorder. She was already on Clonazepam from three weeks of age on but it wasn't cutting it. Sleeping with me solved many problems. She learned how to sleep appropriately, keep her blankets on, stay in bed all night, and trusted that I wouldn't leave her. Therefore she became extremely settled and happy to go to bed at night. Believe me, this didn't happen *overnight*, it was a long, drawn out commitment, and to this day, I still do not sleep with my husband, and I'm completely addicted to cuddling with my angel. I refused to treat her like an animal and put her in a caged bed. She hasn't taken her clothes or diaper off or acted inappropriately since we've changed her sleeping ritual. My husband is dealing with this in a very mature manner. It's more important for our family to get a good night's sleep, and he quite enjoys cuddling with our dog instead (Don't worry! We still manage to enjoy a semi-healthy sex life!).

Sarah has accomplished many things: she walked at three years, she has seven to ten words in her vocabulary, loves to dance in time to the music and clap her hands as of last year. She has learned how to manipulate her entire family. We have a very close, extended family, two aunts and uncles live with their families in our little community. They visit every weekend and are very close to Sarah. She is completely toilet trained at school but not at home—Mommy's fault! She still doesn't want to feed herself—Mommy's fault! I know I have spoiled her too much, and now she expects to be waited on hand and foot.

We share a duplex-type house with my parents living in the other half. It has been a great source of comfort and support for our family. Sarah sees her Nana and Papa every morning. They send her off to school with me and an entourage of two cats and three dogs. The entire community thinks it's quite funny to see Sarah off to school! Nana and Papa are our greatest built-in babysitters. They've saved our lives (and our marriage)! I have special services at home, but only use it in the summer for two afternoons a week so I can get some errands done. She goes to the cottage with my parents twice a year, and we receive a much needed respite break, and we even managed to go to Jamaica this past winter! We couldn't live without them!

She is currently taking 1 mg of Clonazepam and 1.5 mgs of Risperdal. She started on Risperdal approximately four years ago. It's a sedative, antipsychotic, and anti-seizure medication. It was a miracle drug but has since made Sarah gain some unwanted weight around her belly. Now she's on a diet, and we've majorly cut back on her favorite puddings, not an easy feat.

Sarah has had a hard year. She's been hospitalized three times, once with a GI infection and two bouts of pneumonia. These were very scary times, and it's been hard for me to adjust after she's been so ill, but we get over it and go on with life. She has mild seizures that are very controlled, and I realize that we're very lucky that she doesn't have more of a seizure disorder. Sarah had bilateral strabismus repair at the age of two, which has completely straightened her eyes.

When she first came into our lives we thought our lives, as we once knew them, were over. Now we can't imagine our life without her. She has brought our marriage closer and brightens our days with her beautiful smile and wonderful, happy personality. She has been a blessing to our entire family, and we're all proud to call her our *personal Angel*!

ALEX LOVE

This story made its way to me all the way from Australia!
Finding joy in the moments is sometimes so difficult, but
makes life easier to handle when you try.

ENJOY THE MOMENTS

By Ann Love
Mother to Alex

Finding Alex a way to communicate has been very motivating to me. Alex's therapists introduced us to the Picture Exchange Method (PECS). When we first began using PECS, Alex wouldn't look at a picture. It didn't matter if it was in a book, a photo album, etc., he simply wouldn't look, but perseverance and stubborn parenting persevered, and we kept trying. I made giant photo cards of a few familiar foods and other objects that were unfamiliar to Alex. We matched these images up with the objects, and the food. Utilizing the training method described with PECS, Alex very quickly began picking up the card and using it to request what he wanted. He began looking at pictures in shops, in books, in photo albums, as well as the photos on his cards. Using PECS taught Alex how to communicate his wants and needs.

Every day is still a tough day, but now that I am getting more accustomed to them. I realize how much of my strength and my self has gone into my son, to the point where I don't really exist anymore. I know that burnout is not an option. So I am trying to go through a massive transition now. How do you take care of the person who is also the mother of a child with a disability? I don't have that answer yet. Although Alex is my greatest worry, he is also my greatest treatment for worry and stress. Laughing and playing with my son convinces me that we'll make it through if we just remember to enjoy the moments and laugh, a lot.

When I get discouraged, and think, *If only things were different*, I remind myself of the following story and what is really important: let eleven-year-old Connor remind me of what is important. One day Alex and his brother, Connor, were sitting at the table, finishing their lunch when Connor said to me, "Ann, I'm glad Alex has Angelman syndrome."

"Why is that?" I asked.

He said, "Well, if Alex didn't have Angelman syndrome, he would be someone else, and I like Alex."

AUDREY SHORT

I love Tami's story as she discusses that when a child with AS reaches a milestone it is not just a small achievement it is cause for celebration. It gives other AS parents hope that their children can accomplish things as simple as drinking from a sippy cup for the first time or sitting up on their own or taking their first steps.

THE RIGHT THING

By Tami Short
Mother to Audrey

The history leading up to the Angelman syndrome diagnosis was a very stressful time. My daughter Audrey started showing signs of something being wrong shortly after birth. It began with her spitting up a lot with breastfeeding. The spitting up turned into vomiting after feedings, and the frustration I felt with her not being able to hold a feeding in and just being exhausted with having a new baby in the house, and feeling like I was continually trying to feed her while she threw it up every time. By the time she was five weeks old, she had her first hospitalization for the failing to thrive and vomiting. The week prior to this hospitalization we had found out from having an upper GI test that she suffered from reflux. She was placed on reflux medications, but still continued to throw up.

By the age of six weeks, I gave up breastfeeding. It was a very emotional time for me, because I wanted to breastfeed my baby, but she would continue to bring it up. Looking back, I think the problem was that the milk was too thin for her to tolerate. She was placed on a hypoallergenic formula that she tolerated for about a week before starting to throw up again. By the time she was nine weeks old, she had a change in her reflux medication as well as being placed on another hypoallergenic formula. She was hospitalized again due to failure to thrive.

Audrey was transferred to a Children's hospital, because she appeared to have symptoms related to seizures. While at the Children's hospital, various tests were done on her. A variety of specialists also saw her. During this hospital stay, we found out that she was not only dealing with acid reflux, but she also had hypotonic, microcephaly, and strabismus. Looking back, I remember wishfully thinking that all of this was only due to the failure to thrive status, and once that was corrected, everything would correct itself. Thus began our journey of more aggressive testing to figure out what was happening to Audrey.

Audrey was tested for so many things: Lysosomal storage disorders, metabolic disorders, long chain fatty acid disorders, Rett syndrome, Wilson's disease, ataxia telangiectasia, spinal muscular atrophy, etc. I dreaded receiving phone calls about test results, because they always came back *normal*. I reached the point where I'd ask what disorder they were testing her for in order to do an internet search to find out if these tests were related to my daughter's symptoms. After all, I knew my daughter Audrey better than anyone else. By the time she was tested for Rett Syndrome, which occurred around the time she was eight months old, I saw a link to Angelman syndrome and decided to read about it.

It was the first inkling that I had that my daughter might have Angelman syndrome, but she was still young and didn't present with all the characteristic symptoms that were listed. However, looking at photos of other kids with this disorder, I could see some facial similarities and the way the other kids would hold their arms and hands. When Audrey was nine weeks old and in the Children's hospital, a karyotype (normal results), and a FISH test for Prader-Willi syndrome were run on my daughter in addition to some amino acid testing. The results were pending when she was released from the hospital. Unfortunately one of her amino acid results came back exceedingly high, which raised a concern (but fortunately further follow-up testing did not reveal this high level). When I was told about this high amino acid level and the disorder associated with it, I asked about the other tests results, but I did not specify what tests I was asking about. I was told the other tests were *normal*, assuming this meant her karyotype (which was normal), as well as the result of the FISH test (which I would find out months later had never been sent out).

As time went on and more tests were run with normal results, my searches online kept leading me back to Angelman syndrome. Reading about the different genotypes, my guess was that my daughter had the more severe form of Angelman syndrome. As more time went on and my daughter got older, more symptoms would show up that could be associated with Angelman syndrome. At eleven months of age, my daughter was found to be suffering from seizures. I had convinced myself at that point that she had Angelman syndrome. During a clinic visit with Audrey's neurologist, I asked him to test her for Angelman syndrome as I had learned there was more than one test. I asked to have the DNA methylation test done, since it would rule out at least three of the four known genetic forms of Angelman syndrome. The neurologist ordered the test. About three weeks later I was informed that the test results came back *abnormal*. I was happy to receive these results in regards to finally having a test come back showing that something was abnormal. I needed the closure of knowing what was wrong. I no longer had to sit and wonder, *Is my daughter going to walk, talk, feed herself, or is it a neurodegenerative disorder, etc*. We received a positive diagnosis for Angelman syndrome when she was fourteen months old.

There was still the issue on determining what genotype my daughter had. After the abnormal results came back the neurologist ordered a FISH test that showed that Audrey had Angelman syndrome due to a 15q11-13 chromosomal deletion. This was not shocking or upsetting news to me since I had felt months before that my daughter presented with the more severe form of Angelman syndrome.

It has been five years since the diagnosis, and I still have up and down moments. I have moved forward by learning how to work with my daughter on early nonverbal forms of communication, trying to work with her in ways to help her learn, etc. Some of the down moments are dealing with the seizures, the strabismus surgeries my daughter has had to go through, three total. My biggest down moments are whenever I encounter anyone who is exclusive to children with special needs. They are often times rare to see, but you can still encounter them.

With any new child a parent may have, filling out baby books with memorable times when specific milestones are met is something that many of us like to do. Unfortunately, for a child with Angelman syndrome, the milestones are met much later so it can take many, many years for these pages in the baby book to be completed—if completed at all.

Another thing I have noticed is when milestones are finally met for a child with Angelman syndrome, they are not just minor events that you make a notation of and move on, looking for the next milestone or memorable event to happen. No, the milestones that are met for a child with Angelman syndrome are *huge* events to celebrate. Something that seems as simple as, "My child finally learned how to drink out of a straw," or,

"My child pooped on the potty today," may just get a passing yay when other extended family or friends are told, but sharing the exciting news with other parents of kids with Angelman syndrome can result in that child being a *star* for a day as well as giving other parents hope of things that can happen to their children, such as: what did you use to help the child accomplish this, what techniques did you use, what steps did you take on helping your child reach this milestone?

Audrey did not sit up on her own consistently until she was a month away from turning four years old. During a session with her occupational therapist, Audrey was able to get herself into a sitting position several times. I was so happy and couldn't wait to let her show off to her dad. However, once we got home, Audrey wouldn't do it. She wouldn't do it again until ten months later. The day she finally did it again was also the day she started a different antiepileptic medication. I'm sure it was just coincidence as Audrey has since been weaned off this medication, and still gets into a sitting position on her own whenever she wants. This huge milestone for my daughter was finally met on a cold winter morning just a month before she turned four years old.

It took Audrey only three weeks to master phase I of the Picture Exchange Communication System (PECS). It was initially a frustrating time trying to work with her on just picking the picture card up and then trying to get her to hand it to the person she was communicating with. Audrey would become very frustrated with it, because it was as if she felt like she didn't need to hand the picture card to someone to get what she wanted. Instead she would rather take it from the person. We felt it was important for Audrey to learn PECS so that she could initiate communication and continue to build on her nonverbal communication skills. So one afternoon, when I was home alone with her and didn't have the second person needed for phase I of PECS, I decided to try something different. I decided to put the reinforcement item within view, but totally out of Audrey's reach rather than having the reinforcement item between us as she kept trying to reach it, rather than using her PECS card to request the item. Once she saw it was out of her reach, she sat there thinking on how to get the item. She suddenly reached down on her own, picked up the PECS card, and handed it to me. This was such a *huge* event, because it showed us that she didn't need the physical prompting and all the hard and frustrating work we had done over the previous three weeks had paid off. After this Audrey consistently picked up the PECS card on her own, and she would hand it to anyone that had the item she wanted. What was also exciting came just a couple of weeks later when Audrey used what was in her environment and available to her to initiate communication. She saw me eating some candy, and she apparently wanted some as she reached down and picked up an empty candy pack and handed it to me like she did with her PECS card. These were definitely memorable events and huge accomplishments for Audrey.

In order to get Audrey to drink from a straw I took a tip from another parent of a child with Angelman syndrome. Her idea was to use a honey container shaped like a bear and to insert a flexi-straw into the container's lid. I had previously worked with Audrey by squeezing her favorite fluid up through the straw, but she just couldn't suck the fluid up. One night I decided to try something different. Audrey never drinks soda, but on this particular night I decided to try it and see if it would make a difference. I thought the carbonation of the soda would help to keep the fluid in the straw so that she wouldn't have to suck so much. It definitely made a difference, as Audrey took right to it. Not only did she take to drinking the soda, but she also started sucking on the straw. She actually swallowed the fluid *and* she wanted to hold the container on her own. After that one night, she moved on to drinking other fluids out of a straw.

Audrey has for the most part been a quiet little girl with Angelman syndrome. She has done very little babbling, and it seems to come and go. The longest she has held on to a babbling phase has been three months, before it disappeared. Last summer when she was five-and-a-half years old she was doing a lot of babbling, except this time she was associating particular sounds with meaning, such as using *ba-ba-ba* to mean either "binky" or to go outside (I'm assuming her version of saying *bye-bye*). She was making some *goo-goo-good* sounds, and she would stick a *d* sound in there sometimes. I assume she was trying to say, "Good," since she often hears, "Good job," or, "Good girl." However, her first true word was music to my ears... "Mama." It developed over time from just an *mmmm* sound. So for the majority of the summer she would call me *mama* when she needed me or when she was mad at me. Unfortunately I haven't heard her say it since last summer. However, I managed to capture her saying it on videotape several times. It is something I'll always cherish as the first word she spoke. This definitely was one of the most memorable times that I have a date and a word to place in her baby book.

Three of the most frustrating experiences that I have had to deal with involving my child with Angelman syndrome are: finding the diagnosis, visits to the ER, and enrolling in school.

After a year of testing for many disorders, my daughter was finally diagnosed with Angelman syndrome when she was fourteen months old. It wasn't until the DNA methylation test was run on her that we found out what all her symptoms and problems were a result of. It wasn't until she was sixteen months old that the FISH test determined which genetic class of AS she had. Extensive testing began on my daughter when she was nine weeks old. I became so frustrated and so tired of hearing that the results were *normal*—how could all of the tests be normal when my daughter had a huge number of issues going on? In my daughter's case, her diagnosis was not found until the *right* test needed was done. I was so relieved when we finally learned what her diagnosis was. It gave me closure, knowing what specifically was wrong. I needed that closure.

I can thankfully say that in my daughter's six years of life so far, we have only had three visits to the emergency room with her. That's a lot in comparison to the number my other children have had. One frustrating moment came when my daughter was three-and-a-half years old. She had been experiencing a lot of issues with the increase in seizures and the changes in her medication dosages. The more the medication was raised, the worse the seizures got, until my daughter was nearly in a continual state of seizures. She ended up in the ER. The experience in the ER was very frustrating, as the doctor who attended her appeared to have minimal knowledge of seizures in children. He called our neurologist to book an appointment for Audrey in three weeks. This doctor had no experience in dealing with Angelman syndrome but looked it up and read a little about it. He came into the room and told me that I would have to purchase a helmet for Audrey to wear to protect her head from the drop seizures.

My daughter was hooked up to a pulse-ox machine, and every time she would go into a seizure, her oxygen level would drop, sometimes as low as eighty-six. The nurse would just say, "Maybe the machine isn't right, as I'd expect her to have a gray color if it was that low," never bothering to change machines. After spending six hours in the ER and nothing being done, I knew we had to get out of there as my daughter continued having seizures and her oxygen levels were dropping. I finally convinced them to release my daughter, but by the time we reached the neurologist's office it was closed. I called the neurologist the next morning. When he heard what was going on, he advised me to bring her up to the Children's hospital. My daughter was in the hospital for six days. She was on a toxic level from one of her antiepileptic medications. It was three times higher in her than it should have been. She was immediately withdrawn from that medication in the hospital, and a new medication was started. Thankfully seizures of this degree stopped.

My daughter should have gone to Kindergarten this year, but did not. School placement is such a huge issue. I feel my daughter would do best in an inclusive environment in a general education classroom at our local school, while the school feels placing my daughter in a segregated school made up of only severely disabled peers would be my daughter's least restrictive environment. I am told that I need to take it to due process to change the placement; however, who can really afford $25,000-30,000 for due process when there is no guarantee that placement will be changed? Where my daughter should rightfully be able to go to general education classroom (it's her civil right!), I have to prove that my daughter belongs with her peers and deserves to be educated and not just worked with on life skills. Believe it or not, stuff like this is still going on in today's society. I will not lie and say it hasn't been emotionally draining and stressful, as it has been, and I hope another parent never has to deal with what I have.

CADEN GRIFFITH

Thankfully, I have wonderful support from parents of children with AS as well as online support. This story is very special to me as it tells again of a parent advocating for her child, wanting the community to know her child and not be afraid to ask about him and get to know him.

HE LOVES IN A HARD WAY, BUT HE IS ALL LOVE

By Elisha Griffith
Mother to Caden

I met Caden on June 23, 2003. I had the usual anxiety… what will he look like, what will his personality be, and what will our future be? We got off to a rocky start, him not too sure about me, and me very frustrated with him. He tested me nonstop the first few weeks to see if I would give up on him. Then slowly over the next several months he began to soften a bit. I received a few smiles between the frowns, and he allowed slightly more touching to build up tolerance and trust. I wasn't sure that I felt much for him, but I saw the pain he endured, and I had pity on him. I watched as he struggled to make sense of his life. I ached inside when I saw the pain on his face. After about two weeks, we started supplementing him with formula, because he was not gaining weight appropriately. We tried every kind of formula out there, but he was not gaining enough weight. At around two months he was diagnosed with reflux. When he was six months old we noticed a delay in his development. It wasn't until he reached nine months of age that we were referred to several specialists. Caden was hospitalized and was put through a gamut of tests, with nothing out of the ordinary showing up. The gastro doctor put him on Pediasure, which helped with his low weight. The neurologist said he would catch up developmentally now that he was gaining weight, but to come and see him when Caden was eighteen months old if things didn't improve.

That was May of 2004. In July, we went in for Caden's one-year appointment, in which he got an A+ for catching up on his weight, Dr. Patyrak was very proud. However, for about a week, Caden's brother, Colebin, had been urinating frequently, was moody, and thinning out. At the same appointment, he was tested and hospitalized for diabetes. This blew us away, since he was always so healthy. Pretty soon we were educated on taking care of a child with diabetes. Colebin could live a very normal life. It wouldn't always be easy, but promising for the future. This was a difficult time for our family. Our focus was then again turned toward Caden in August. He was still behind physically, which didn't bother me nearly as much as what I was seeing in the cognitive area. I kept thinking and feeling like there wasn't something right about how he handled himself and reacted to situations. So the search continued for what was going on with him.

At this point the search was more difficult, because the fight was not only to find the problem, but also to convince others that there was something to find. I didn't want to wait until eighteen months to see the neurologist again. I was losing precious developmental months by waiting. I searched the Internet looking for anything, but kept coming up with nothing. I flew with Caden to a physical pherapist in Conroe to have an evaluation done. She was supposed to be very keen in sensing problems. Although I didn't get any answers from her, I did get some ideas on where to start looking. I finally felt like I was doing something. She said to first have his ears tested, and if his ears were fine, to go immediately to the neurologist. Her main concern was that he wasn't verbalizing anything. We did have his ears tested and tested and tested. We finally got approval for tubes to be put in, in October of 2004. A test after the tubes were put in came back inconclusive, which made us think there may still be a problem with his hearing. I knew that he could hear a little, because he responded to my voice. I was at my wit's end trying to figure it out and trying to decide if I was just crazy and he was fine. The only area we had not covered was his head. I asked Dr. Patyrak to do a head exam, which he kindly agreed to, although I think he was skeptical himself. After a grueling ordeal of trying to schedule the MRI, we were called the week of Thanksgiving and told that we could do it on that Friday. Although very inconvenient, we did the MRI, and it came back *normal*. On the Sunday after Thanksgiving, I had coffee with a good friend of mine,

Hollie. She had been to Oklahoma in October to visit a friend of hers. For some reason Caden's developmental delay came up in their conversation. Her friend asked if he was happy all the time. Hollie answered yes. Her friend told her to have us look into Angel Syndrome. I was skeptical, just because everything we had tested for had come back *negative*. However, when I got home I did a search and found Angelman Syndrome. It nailed Caden. There were some things that Caden didn't have, which made us wonder if this was truly what he had. I printed off what I had read and sent them to Dr. Patyrak that Monday. A week later they tested Caden for Angelman syndrome. Originally they said it would take two weeks, but later changed it to four weeks. At four weeks, I called to see if the results were in. Dr. Patyrak called back immediately with a positive result. That was January 2, 2005. My heart slowly began to build up love that would become an overflowing fountain. At a year-and-a-half we got our answer. We were intended to spend the rest of our lives together. The testing was over, the early growing pains were almost through. Our roles started to be defined: I would care for him, and he would be my teacher.

By this point we were just happy to have the answer to the question we had searched nine months for. It was several months later that it really sunk in, and I think it's still sinking. When we hit new challenges with Colebin or Caden, it becomes more of a reality.

My state of mind about all this is amazing to me. I know that it is the power of God working. I would not be able to handle these things without the confidence that God is taking care of all things.

After the word started getting out about Caden's diagnosis, we received numerous calls and cards of thoughts, prayers, and gift certificates to restaurants. One woman called and offered to watch the boys one morning. I needed some time to myself more than anything in those first weeks in January. A class at church takes up donations and we were the receivers of those donations twice. One family donated a car to us. We received several personal monetary donations. A friend left a basket of goodies on my porch when she knew I was having a rough time. Another friend gave me the precious gift of *my time*, scrapbooking. I assume there were numerous people who made it possible for Mike, Colebin, and I to go on a Diabetic Camp Cruise in June. I received a scholarship, after having been turned down originally, to attend a conference in California on Angelman syndrome. To this same conference, my airline ticket was paid for. Our car broke down, and it was going to cost a large sum to fix. We were called and told to pick up the car; it was fixed and paid for. My friends have been right by my side, supporting me and checking on me frequently. Everytime one of the boys is in the hospital, I can count on numerous visits and calls. I can't even begin to name all the areas in which our parents have helped us. I continue to feel so overwhelmed with the amount of love and support we have from all our family and friends. I feel very sad for people who do not have what we have been increasingly blessed with. I have no doubt that God has good intentions for the trials that we face. I've learned so much this past year educationally, emotionally, and spiritually. I would never have learned these things if it weren't for the experiences we have had. We do have some challenges ahead of us, but because of all of you, we have the support to conquer those challenges. Colebin will develop characteristics that he wouldn't have had otherwise by having to handle his diabetes. Not to mention that it guarantees him somewhat equal attention from his parents. Caden, although not the *normal* child everyone thinks they are going to have, is a lesson all by himself. Don't get me wrong, I feel sorry for myself some days when I'm covered in slobber, refluxed food, my hair has the teased effect after being spit up in and pulled, my waist band is stretched out from Caden standing on it all day and all I've done all day is clean up one mess after another. However, it only takes two seconds of looking at his smiling face to forget all the frustration. You are a pretty sour individual if you don't find yourself smiling when you see Caden. He loves in a hard way, but he is all love. The greatest commandment is to love.

It has been almost four years, and Caden and I share a thousand hugs a week and ten thousand kisses. He has brought more unconditional love to my life than any I've ever known. My face lights up the moment I see him whether it's been seconds, minutes, or days. His smile reaches truly as far as the east is from the west. If ever there were a portrait for God's love, it would be the smile on his face. He sees no color, no race, no gender, no handicap, no immorality, or sin. He just loves people. He is my son, and he has Angelman syndrome. Now almost four, his first two years of life were hard with battles of health issues and physical ailments. But today he is a fun-loving boy that just makes you grin. And I'm happy to spend the rest of my life smiling with him.

ADAM JAMES SPROW

*I am fortunate enough to know Elke and Adam personally.
Elke is very proactive with her son, always trying to figure
out what he wants or needs: trying to get him to 'use his
words' and figuring out age appropriate activities that he
can join in with his peers. It is a pleasure to know them and
their family.*

LIFE ACCORDING TO ADAM

By Elke Sprow
Mother to Adam

Adam has Angelman syndrome. He is the second of
our four children and the only boy.

When my first child, Hannah, was two years old, we
decided to try for another child. I remember the day I
got pregnant and the day I found out I was pregnant.
It was just one of those things; you know what you
know, part of a grand design that is beyond yourself.
This child, this little boy that was growing inside me,
was meant to be. I knew when I got the pregnancy test
result that we would have a boy, there was no doubt
at all in my mind. I knew his name would be Adam.
I knew he would be blond and beautiful. All of this
turned out to be true!

What I couldn't know was that he would be born with a genetic aberration that would change our lives. When I was eleven weeks pregnant, I had what is called a *level two ultrasound*. The technicians take a special measurement called a *nuchal fold transclucency screening*, where the amount of fluid on the back of the baby's neck is measured. It is a common test today and can indicate a chromosomal abnormality. Not definitively, but it can suggest a need for further testing.

Adam's test was abnormal. As we watched the little boy kick and suck his thumb on the ultrasound screen, I knew that we were going to have this child no matter what. Adam was born on All Saints Day, November 1, 2004. It was fitting that we had an Angel even then. When Adam was born, he looked and seemed quite normal, despite having feeding and sleep issues.

However, he was a healthy little guy: flirty, lovable, a true joy. It wasn't until Adam was around seven months of age that I started to sense that something wasn't right. After taking him to five different pediatricians, we finally walked into an office in Napa, California, and said, "Dr. Meyers, something is just not right, please help." The doctor mentioned that he had other patients in his clinic with low tone like Adam, and so he tested Adam for something called Prader Willi syndrome. It was a shock when we were told, a short time later, that he had Prader Willi. With a crash course in genetics from the Internet, we discovered that Prader Willi had a sister syndrome, called Angelman syndrome. The two syndromes only differed in the discovery process, with the error for Prader Willi occurring on the paternal chromosome and the error for Angelman syndrome occurring on the maternal chromosome. One week after the first incorrect diagnosis of Prader Willi, we finally had the correct one: Adam was deletion positive for Angelman syndrome.

In the course of a month, we went from believing we had a rather slow but normal little boy, to the reality of a lifelong, rather severe, neurological disability, affecting this baby we loved so much. We were devastated. It was one of the only times in my marriage that I have seen my husband shed tears. He cried for two weeks while I walked around in a fog, thinking, *What the heck happened and would someone please stop this train so that I could get off?*

Good sense finally kicked in, and we came to terms with needing to understand the reality we were handed. I am a person of science, so I leaned on that. My husband is more existential than me and relied on his faith. Together, we moved forward with our son, our daughter, and our lives.

Since that time, we have two more little girls and a world of knowledge under our belts on Angelman syndrome. We found that yes indeed, science could help, and what science couldn't help with, faith could. God has given us this incredible soul to guide through life, and we are committed to doing just that in the very best ways we can. This includes a routine of therapeutic pharmaceuticals, like levodopa, that enhance Adam's ability to learn and to move. It also includes lots of hugs, firm discipline (the teaching kind, not the corporal punishment kind), lots social and sensory input, heaps of patience on our parts, and a foundation of faith that is nurtured daily in our homes and weekly in our church, for the good of our entire family.

It isn't always easy, and it is often a whole lot of no fun, but there is no way I would trade this little boy for anything, in this universe or the next. He has shown me, daily a little bit of his world, and daily, I show him a little bit of mine. We meet in the middle, with each of us a better person for the whole experience.

Adam is special, yes. He runs, rides bike, rides horse, climbs like a monkey, and is a general daredevil. He is an intrepid explorer, much to our dismay sometimes, and makes a mess like nobody's business. I am certain he has a future job in consumer product testing, because if something can stand up to Adam's busy hands, you can be sure it will last. He loves to help mow the lawn, do laundry, vacuum, and help me make apple pie. He loves to help his dad paint building projects, and he dearly loves playing with his sisters and friends. I swear that Adam walks with one hand in this world and the other hand firmly tucked in God's. For how else can one explain the joy and love that he exhibits throughout the day, every day?

He is a typical boy in many ways, such as loving to play ballgames of all kinds, playing in the mud, pretending to build with his play tools, and playing trucks and trains. He loves airplanes and elevators and anything to do with getting wet. When he is unhappy, he is not shy about letting us know it. He can throw a tantrum like my other children, and we deal with it the same as we do with our other children. We always teach manners and insist on following the household rules no matter what. Shoes have to be put in the proper place, spoons go in the sink, and no, no child is allowed to get away with whatever they want, including Adam. In many ways, treating him like there is nothing at issue with him has allowed us, as a family, to be more *normal*. Not a bad deal and great for our collective sanity.

Adam has taught us many things, and the journey is still young. We have a long way to go, I hope. Whatever the future holds, I am immensely thankful and grateful that God has chosen to grant us this time with this special soul. We will do our part to love him and give him the tools he needs for the best quality life he can achieve, and he will do his part to give us a lifetime of smiles and laughter and messes. While we are often perplexed and tired, we are also full to the brim with Adam's love and hugs and kisses. There will never, ever, be a boring day with Adam.

KYLEE KOHLER

This story struck from the onset. I love when people accept their life and live it to the fullest.

UTTER CUTENESS

By Sylvia Kohler
Mother to Kylee

So many years, so many experiences, but our initial introduction to other Angelman families during the conference in Orlando, Florida, in 1993, just after Kylee got diagnosed, was certainly memorable and a moment of great relief. As Kylee had not been diagnosed until she was ten, I had been able to adjust to the shock and despair of having a child with disabilities, but not knowing exactly what was wrong and not finding answers to her sleep problems and other issues most particularly frustrated me. Many (including her Neurologist whom I persuaded to give her the blood test for AS), said I was just searching for a label. The sense of wanting to find a home to the answers to my many questions—and yes, finding other children who did not sleep at night—was profound. I remember arriving at the hotel where the conference was being held at about ten at night. Driving in I saw a lot of the kids in the pool, and I laughed out loud, and knew we belonged, and that we had finally found our home. And of course we went to join them!

Kylee continues to surprise me with her growing level of comprehension over the years. She will follow through in commands that I have never asked her to do before, and then she will throw me that very cute Angel smile, which so clearly says, "Gotcha," as she senses I fell into that trap of disbelief yet again. She truly knows so much more than we give her credit for. I never cease to marvel at those moments of her figuring things out. I remember one day close to lunch telling her to go downstairs to play with her beanies. When I finally got down there, she had the fridge door open, had pulled out her cheeses, and was eating one of her yogurts... with a fork, but that hardly matters. She was eating it just fine, and yes, really laughing at me at the same time! It was truly memorable!

Kylee's biggest challenge—I think in large part, stemming from her great stubbornness—is toilet training. She absolutely refuses to sit on the toilet for me, although in younger years we did have some successes. I know that she understands the concept of toilet training, but has decided she doesn't like it and so be it. I remember one day after a tub she had that look; yes, she needed to go. I tried to get her to sit on the toilet, but her resistance was strong, and she kept pointing to her room where the diapers were. Well, of course she won that fight, headed for her room, gave me a diaper, and as soon as it was on, did her business!

I will say that I am happy that my mom and dad—and Kylee's dad and his family as well—never had a problem accepting Kylee for who she is. I think her utter cuteness and coy ways won us over, and she has all of us wrapped around her little finger! We have always loved her and accepted her, even at some of the most trying times, and that is worth a lot. And importantly for her, she knows she is loved unconditionally (With a lot of attempts at behavior management thrown in too!).

Thankfully, good friends to vent to—and party with—have helped me tremendously over the years... plus a sense of the absurd thrown into the mix as well. Obviously, on emergency runs to the hospital, which were terrifying to me, their support was unquestioned.

MARY CATE (CATIE) WILES

This proves that we do have very special children.

TRULY AN ANGEL

By Mary Susanne Cato
Mother to Catie

Catie has always been a joy to us. In a home full of kids, most of them teens, you learn to appreciate a child who is so full of love and affection.

When Catie was about six or seven, we were at the hospital lab waiting to get her blood drawn (again). A lady and her husband came in, and since the waiting room was crowded, stood beside Catie. The lady was crying softly, and her husband kept hugging her. I suddenly realized that Catie had reached up from her tiny wheelchair and was holding this woman's free hand. I quickly grabbed Catie's hand away and murmured an apology. I was so embarrassed. The lady said, "No it's okay." They went before we did, and when they came out the lady came up to me and said, "I got some bad news today and was crying because I was feeling sorry for myself. When your little angel grabbed my hand I felt like everything was going to be okay. You really have a special child." From that day on I knew Catie was truly an Angel.

Catie's preschool teacher was the one who guessed she had Angelman syndrome. When I brought this up to her neurologist, he was adamant that she did not have it. He swore he knew more about it than most doctors, and he would of diagnosed it himself if she had it. He did agree to test her for it. A few months later on a Sunday night I got a phone call from the neurologist. He said, "I knew it, she does have Angelman syndrome. I just knew she did!" It was hard not to laugh out loud!

JUSTIN STADNYK

An Angel who talks and rides a bike? Who knew!

A CHALLENGING LIFESTYLE

By Debra Stadnyk
Mother to Justin

Our most cherished experience with Justin is his ability to say, "Mama," which means, "Mom," and "Dad."

When Justin was two years old he contracted severe pneumonia, which developed into empyema. As a result he needed a thoracotomy and chest tubes, and then he had a severe allergic reaction to a group of antibiotics that caused a severe illness.(he looked like a thousand bees had stung him and then been dropped into boiling water).

Justin and his younger brother, Carter are best friends. What a true blessing! Justin's best therapist is Carter, because he wants to imitate him and do all the same activities in play.

Justin was completely potty-trained by the age of six. I have a tip that helped us get to this point. Try putting a wet piece of toilet paper on your child's privates when sitting on the potty. I made it wet so it stuck and gave a sensory cue to help the brain signal where to squeeze the muscles. This is only my theory, but it worked like a charm for Justin.

Our biggest challenge with Justin is communication. Thankfully, our family is very accepting and involved in giving us respite care when we really need it. The challenge of raising a child with Angelman syndrome has helped our family and friends learn better acceptance and understanding of people with disabilities.

Exercise gave me more energy and better coping abilities on a regular basis. It is a challenging lifestyle, and as parents of an Angel, there is very little we can control, like the lack of sleep, the constant hands-on supervision of endless energy, various health issues, and all the appointments that go along with raising a child with a disability.

But the one thing that I can do is improve my physical health and, in doing so, it improves my energy level and my ability to handle stress. Sometimes it is easier said than done. I have often gone for months of not exercising regularly (after an illness, busy schedule, etc). But when I do exercise, I have noticed a huge improvement in my mental and emotional well-being.

KENT (GRAHAM) DROVER

One evening shortly after I had my letters requesting stories on AS published in the ASF and CASS newsletters, there was a phone call. My husband answered the phone and looked puzzled as he passed me the phone. It was Louise Drover. Her East Canadian accent was too much for my husband. I spoke to this lovely woman about her son Graham and my book effort for nearly an hour. It was very uplifting and special to me to hear her gush about her beloved son and hear her excitement about the book.

THE SPARKLE
IN MY LIFE

By Louise Drover
Mother to Graham

Graham Kent Drover was born on March 23, 1985. He was the third child born to John and Louise Drover of Blaketown, Newfoundland, Canada.

It was a beautiful crystal morning as we traveled the highway to the nearby city of St. John's. The glitter on the trees, caused by the freezing rain the night before, made the appearance of heavenly angels. I knew that that day I would give birth to my baby. Little did I know how special this child was going to be.

Just like the trees that sparkled that morning along the Trans Canada Highway, each with their angelic glow, so too would my son be the sparkle in my life. He would have an angelic glow that would touch the hearts of all he met along his life's highway. Today I would have an "Angel Child".

Graham was a small wiggly ragdoll, like baby. He cried a lot. He spit up a lot. He had bowel problems. He was hospitalized for suffering from malnutrition. This was caused by his digestive problems. We changed his diet to skim milk, prune juice, and homemade baby foods. He soon became well and strong.

At the age of two he still didn't walk and, although infant walkers were labeled as unsafe at the time, I found an old one and boy could he go. His legs got stronger, and he started to walk. Also at the age of two years, it was discovered that Graham had vision problems. This was corrected with surgery and glasses.

We were sure everything would be okay now. He was walking, he could see fine, and was eating well. What else could go wrong? Our baby was going to grow into a fine young man.

Then came the worst day of our lives. We went to see a child neurologist, and on our very first visit his exact words were, "Your baby is not normal, just look at him, he doesn't even look normal." Those were the worst words I had ever heard. I cried all the way home and for months after.

So many thoughts and questions ran through my mind. I would think, *This is not the baby I carried to the doctor that day. My baby was not handicapped. Where is my baby? What went wrong? Was it my fault? How can I go on? What will I do? Can anyone make him better?*

Two things happened to change my feelings. My daughter Betty-Lou, who was thirteen years old at the time, saw me crying and said to me, "Mom, how can you cry so much when Graham is so happy?" Then one morning I awoke to find my husband next to Graham's crib sobbing and crying. Something had to change. It was then that I said, "Now Mom, you have to stop this. You have a husband and three children to care for, and all this self-pity is doing nothing for your situation." It was at that moment that I knew Graham was going to live the best life he could and that our whole family was going to be okay. It was going to start right now.

My wedding vows from fourteen years earlier rang strong in my mind. For better, for worse, for richer, for poorer, in sickness, and in health. Although our lives seemed to lean toward the worse, poorer, and sickness part, there was still lots of love, and this family would flourish on love. I just knew it would.

Our son Colin was around eleven years old at this time, and he sure loved his little brother. At times his young friends would sometimes tease him about Graham being different. As a result one of his buddies got thrown into the nearby pond. As they all matured they came to accept Graham and saw him as a good little buddy. No one else made fun of Graham after the pond incident!

Graham started having seizures when he was seven. This was a difficult time. The seizures began to settle down by the time he reached his teenage years. Now at the age of twenty-two there haven't been any seizures for years. Thank God for Graham's gift of medication.

Something wonderful did happen during one of his seizures. His eyesight corrected itself. There will be no more surgery or glasses. His vision is perfect today.

Graham's medication now consists of Depekane (for seizures), Sulcrate (for digestive problem), and Melatonin (for sleep his disorder). He is quite healthy and doing well. He is doing so well, in fact, that the last time he saw his neurologist he asked Graham, "Do you like birthday parties?" Graham responded by clapping his hands and blowing on his finger. "Good," said Dr. Hall, "you will probably have a hundred of them!"

Life with Graham has had its ups and downs. We have had some wonderful memories to downright scary ones, and lots, and lots of funny ones. Our best memory lasted a full week. In November of 2002, our whole family went to Disney World, which was sponsored by The Sunshine Foundation. What an experience for this low-income family. What a magical time. We will never forget our once-in-a-lifetime trip. The glow and excitement on Graham's face was our greatest thrill, and that excelled everything else for us. We will never forget the excited squeals, with clapping and flapping of his hands as so many Disney characters stepped out of the parade to personally speak to him.

It was a trip of a lifetime. We know that Graham still remembers the trip, because when he looks at the photos of our trip or sees Disneyworld on the TV, he becomes very excited.

Graham has caused our hearts to pound with fear many times, but the scariest time was at a mall in St. John's, Newfoundland. I was watching him from inside an office window as Graham slowly edged his way out of the office and stood beside the glass door to watch the people pass. As I was watching, a strange man passed him and patted him on the head. He then went to an ATM machine and motioned for Graham to come over. Graham quickly went to his side, and as I approached the stranger, he was whispering something in Graham's ear. The man became noticeably upset when I appeared on the scene. I was shaking as we went back to the safety of the office where my husband was doing some business.

My suspicions were confirmed a week later when that very man appeared on the local news. I thank God that I was closely watching Graham, and I got to my baby just in time. That same year at a smaller mall I lost Graham. I turned around, and he was gone. I ran through the mall with the thoughts of the past summer's horrific ordeal still fresh in my mind, and I panicked. I ran to the Salvation Army kettle volunteers at the entrance and said, "I can't find Graham, don't let him out." An announcement was made over the PA system. Two teenage girls had found Graham and brought him to the customer service desk. When we got to him, he was devouring a box of chocolates. He had chocolate drool from his chin to his waist. The lovely young ladies were dressed to the nines in beautiful white blouses, and they were holding Graham at arms length. It was then that a very disturbing thought entered my head. *Would we claim him or just walk away as if we didn't know him.* But of course we claimed him; we loved him, chocolate, drool, and all.

Life with Graham has not been all smooth sailing. I have sailed through some very rough water and sometimes feel as if I am not going to make it. The calm waters always seem to return again to Newfoundland Bay, but as sure as the calm waters return, so do the rough waters. I have often been told to live one day at a time, but sometimes a day is too long, so I try to get through the next few minutes. Between the Graham's squeals and his foot stomping, which he does when he doesn't get his own way, there is such a perfect peace. A beautiful quiet rests.

Graham has strengthened me with a richer love and a stronger faith. He has taught me to accept certain things and to do the best I can with everyday. We all love him very much, and he is the best thing that has ever happened to us. What would I do without Graham?

Graham's greatest accomplishment is to have lived a good life with lots of friends, to be accepted as a valued member of his community. Everyone knows him, and he is very popular. He has a wonderful respite worker, Florence, who includes him in everything she does. Everyone loves Graham.

Some things are hard to think about, but we will care for him as long as we can. But someday we have to accept the fact that this earthly angel will become a heavenly angel at which time "Those who cannot speak will shout for joy" (Isaiah 35:5 KJV).

LANGUAGE OF OUR ANGELS

To one who knows an Angel this poem says it all.

By Kathleen Marie Short
Aunt to an Angel

I bite
I pinch
I slap
I stomp
I whine
I'm communicating.
Don't you hear me?
My language is not words.
God gave me something else.
He gave you words.
He also gave you empathy,
So that you could better understand me.
It's our bridge.
Please use it to connect us.
And you will know, that when I bite,
I love you so much I want to eat you all up.
I pinch so hard because my emotions cannot contain
    themselves
So they must squeeze through my fingers.
My pats of endearment express themselves as slaps.
My stomps keep me grounded
Giving my frustration back to Mother Earth.

And most important of all, my whining, as you call it,
Is my sincerest form of communicating with my lack
of words,
For the deep sadness and disappointment I feel in
how much we both are missing.
I'm reaching out in the best way I know how
Using the only real language we both understand

Love
Aunt Kathleen

ELENA PALOMORES

I couldn't hold back my excitement from receiving an email with a submission all the way from Spain! We were able to email a couple of times and the love Maria shares for her daughter and her family shone through.

WITH LOVE
AND A SENSE OF HUMOR
ALL IS POSSIBLE

By Maria Galan
Mother to Elena

I remember, with great pleasure, the tenderest moments in Elena's life; my husband and I had just returned home from the hospital with our third child. When Elena saw him for the first time, he was crying. All of a sudden she dove under the couch and retrieved a little piece of paper that she carefully placed on her new baby brother. She gave him her beloved treasure—a little piece of paper.

When Elena was three years old, she woke us up in the middle of the night, crying. Soon her crying turned to vomiting. Suddenly a piece of hard plastic, seven centimeters long, appeared in her mouth. She was in the hospital for two weeks, because the plastic had damaged her throat and esophagus.

Elena was the third child to be diagnosed with Angelman syndrome in Spain and the first Angelman child in my area. This was one of the worst experiences of our whole lives, getting this diagnosis. My family has always been close to us, and they love Elena. My mother and Elena love each other very much. I think Elena loves her more than me!

In my experience, the first moments of the diagnosis are the worst, because your whole world feels like it has fallen away under your feet. When she had all of her therapies and doctor appointments organized, with the help of my family, I finally felt like my life could move forward.

I find myself wondering what will happen to my child when she gets older, what will happen to her when we are not around. How will she feel when we are gone?

When you have a *special* child in your family, the whole family is special for many reasons. In our family there were so many places we couldn't go because of Elena. For example, it was not possible for the whole family to go to the cinema, because Elena was always making noises or yelling. Fortunately because of Elena, my other children have become more understanding and patient with other children. My children are the first to befriend new students at school and offer their friendship.

I think Elena has *enriched* our whole family. Her having Angelman syndrome has allowed us to learn things that we may not have learned otherwise. That is the best part of having Angelman syndrome be a part of our lives.

We believe you can only cope with a *special* child in your family if your family is united. One day you are supporting your husband, and one day he is supporting you.

We always taught our children that Elena is a very important member of our family. When Elena would pull our youngest daughters hair I would always say, "Cristina you must be happy and honored, because Elena is saying, 'I love you Cristina.'" Of course this is very difficult for a baby to understand, but little by little, and with love and a sense of humor, *all* is possible.

KATIE KAMPSCHNEIDER

I love this story of working together as a family to care for Katie so that no one person does it alone. They all get to share in the blessing of caring for someone special.

WE ARE ALL DOING OUR SHARE

By Mary Jo Kampschneider
Mother to Katie

While we were attending an Angelman Conference in Colorado, Katie was pushing the stroller that her two-year-old brother Jake was riding in. Some people walking by commented that our Angel was doing very well, sitting up so straight in the stroller. They were shocked to hear that Katie was the Angel and not her brother. The smallest positive comment helped us to establish our goals of helping Katie be the best she could be and to blend in to the community.

When Katie was about five years old we were very open to natural remedies to enhance Katie's life. We got involved with Chinese herbs. During the difficult times of sleep deprivation and hard-to-control laughter, we worked on getting Katie's body in balance. Through all the research we did we became very confident about starting our daughter on Chinese herbs. After a few weeks on the herbs we started to see improvement with Katie's sleep and behaviors. This was great until we realized that giving our daughter unknown ingredients may not be in her best interest. When she turned eight she began puberty. We saw an endocrinologist, which after several tests, determined that her prepuberty was not associated with the herbs at all. It was just her time to start. We were so relieved that we didn't contribute toward her early start. From this experience we learned to always check with our doctor or to find a doctor who has knowledge about administration of nonmedicinal remedies.

Katie has mastered so many things. She is toilet trained, she has a very strong understanding of all conversation, she sleeps in a queen-size bed all by herself, and she has mastered her augmentative device. With this device she has shown us that she believes in and acknowledges God.

The very first time Katie went on a merry-go-round, she loved it! Her mouth was open so wide, and the look on her face was pure happiness. We will always cherish this memory.

Katie's biggest challenge to date is social interaction. She is very shy. When she is in socially uncomfortable situations, she resorts to poor conduct and laughter to help her escape from the situation. Her behavior will escalate until she is removed. As a result, it is very hard for her to make friends and interact with others in different situations and settings.

My extended family is very supportive. They have helped us through extremely difficult times. They continue to be very good listeners, which help when we need to problem solve. Recognizing that there is an education process of learning how to give respite care has been a challenge for them, which has been hard for us.

Katie has brought us all closer to God. She has strengthened our compassion for people and has helped us focus on trying to be nonjudgmental toward others. Katie has definitely brought out our creativity as a family. I can't even begin to express how much Katie has helped her brothers grow into such caring individuals. At the ages of ten and twelve they show so much maturity through their care, love, and protection that they demonstrate to others and to Katie. Through their experiences with Katie and the love they have shown her, I am certain they will be outstanding fathers.

I give my hard times to God, which makes everything do-able. Our goal as a family is to attempt to limit the *tough* days. We have productive family meetings to discuss issues and problem solve together, which helps each of us feel like we are contributing. We keep a journal of the solutions we come up with and then work together on resolving problems. One of the things that we needed to problem solve as a family was meal preparation. It is very difficult to prepare a meal with Katie around, because she gets into everything. The solution we came up with is that the boys take turns interacting with Katie to keep her busy while I get the meal ready.

This has worked out nicely. We have all agreed to it, and we are all doing our share.

KILEY JOY WILLIAMS

Sitting in my first Angelman Syndrome conference, feeling very vulnerable, I saw the most adorable couple: Gini and James Williams. We became fast friends and had several great talks together. It was during one of our talks that she mentioned to me how on every Tuesday of every week, they pray for Kiley and other children that need miracles in their lives. She said that they would like to add Conrad to that list. I have felt those prayers and I have seen miracles.

CHOOSING JOY

By Gini Williams

We will never forget December 3, 2005.

I was on my way to the mall to purchase a last minute gift for my husband's business Christmas party, which was scheduled to start in less than an hour.

I pulled in to a parking space outside Macy's with an adrenaline rush as I was in a hurry to get in and wrestle the crowds for a quick purchase and escape.

I shuffled to answer my cell phone as I unfastened my seatbelt and opened the car door.

An unfamiliar number; I paused and slipped back into my seat, took a deep breath, and prepared to answer.

Was this the call I had been anxiously awaiting? Would this be the answer to so many questions? Certainly, it would be the close of a frustrating and confusing chapter of questions and uncertainty in our lives. I hoped. And, I feared.

Five weeks earlier, we found out we were pregnant! What Joy! Another baby!

Upon learning this news, Kiley Joy's pediatric neurologist suggested we make an appointment at the genetics center to inquire for concluding answers to the increasing delay challenging our firstborn baby girl.

Anyone who has children understands the immense amount of overwhelming joy, excitement, and anticipation surrounding the birth of their firstborn baby. There is an emotion so natural and so equally supernatural that it is almost indescribable.

Immediate dreams and desires and goals are inspired. There is instant pride, joy, and unconditional love formed the moment you first see and hold your newborn child.

We were no different. James and I met in high school when we were fifteen and seventeen years old. We dated for six years, through high school and college. We were married at the very young age of twenty and twenty-two.

We were very excited to start our family together a few short, three, years later.

September 27, 2004. After six short hours of labor we held our sweet angel, Kiley Joy Williams, our first-born baby girl, weighing, 5 lbs. 6 oz. and 17 inches long. Her hair was long and golden blonde. With deep, bright, blue eyes, she was glowing!

My sister said that she looked like Sunshine!

She was our baby girl—Daddy's little girl, Mommy's best friend, pink walls, bracelets, hairbows, butterfly kisses, learning to ride a bike, throw a ball, ballet lessons, dancing with Daddy, reading bedtime stories with Mommy, learning about Jesus, a sweet little voice singing, "Jesus loves me," a solo in the Christmas play, homecoming queen, a college degree, a wedding, grandchildren…

We were inundated with rapidly forming dreams and goals and visions for our life with this precious little gift! The excitement grew and doubled each passing day.

We fell in love with her.

At the gentle age of fourteen months, I took Kiley Joy for a blood test at the genetics center. I shared every concern with the doctor. She listened attentively and graciously.

What caught her interest most was my explanation of this completely happy little girl: a sweet angel baby that literally *never* ever cried. In fact, in her twelve, short months of life, we hadn't seen a single tear fall from her eyes. Kiley Joy was always happy and content and smiling and laughing.

She really was sunshine!

I left the office with a *clinical diagnosis* of Angelman syndrome, only to have it be confirmed later by tests. I had no idea what to expect. I had never heard of Angelman syndrome. I certainly didn't expect to discover the extent of information waiting for me at home as I studied the Internet desperately seeking answers.

I read information about many different children with this same diagnosis and the constant challenge and battles that they face everyday. I read of the different disabilities and handicaps and developmental delays affecting these children. Doctor's warned us "not to expect to see her walk or to talk."

With each new article, doctor report, or personal story I discovered, I grew fearful and sad.

For five weeks I read and studied and compared and contrasted my precious baby Kiley Joy to the statistics and facts online.

That December day, I slipped back into my seat and answered my cell phone.

I held my breath through the initial phone etiquette and greeting formalities. The voice on the other end said, "Mrs. Williams, the test results have confirmed positive for Angelman syndrome. You will need to call to make an appointment with the genetics counselor at your earliest convenience."

I managed a fragile, "Thank you." And the call ended.

I heard the answer I had feared.

The world started spinning. Outside the windows of my car, everything seemed gray and curiously silent, yet, increasingly loud.

I cried. I cried so hard. I remember shaking and feeling so very weak.

To this day, I don't remember the drive home. I was emotionally and mentally absent from the world. I managed a phone call to my husband telling him the news.

The next thing that I recall was sitting on the end seat of our couch in our living room, crying. I remember staring at the wall straight ahead of me.

I have a vague memory of my brother kneeling beside the couch, holding my hands. My sister sat across from me and my husband beside me. There were many family members in the room. Each face streamed with tears at the realization of this heartbreak.

After all, our dreams and desires for her little life were slipping away with each passing moment of realization.

I don't remember much of anything after that night of crying on our couch.

I don't remember a single day for the next three months of life. It's as if life was passing me by, and I was too full of disappointment, grief, heartbreak, and broken dreams to notice anything.

I was sad, broken, and afraid.

I was sad everyday.

I remember waking up one morning and thinking to myself, *I don't want to feel sad like this every day for the rest of my life. I don't want my family and friends to be sad for me.* I remember thinking, *Gini, you have a choice. You can lie in bed and be sad for the rest of your time here on Earth, or you can get up and try to be happy.*

My family and I do not believe that happiness is something that happens to us.

We have learned that happiness is a decision and a choice.

I had no idea how to be happy. I remember having to consciously make the mental effort to upright my body to the edge of my bed. I had to physically lift my legs to the ground and with all the strength left in my arms, push off the mattress in order to stand up. I remember standing at the side of my bed and not knowing what to do next.

I was so confused. I didn't know how to be happy. I had lost my joy.

I made myself walk to the bathroom, look in the mirror, and brush my teeth and my hair. Not because I felt like it, but because it was what I knew one was *supposed* to do in the morning to get ready for the day.

Morning after morning, I woke up and challenged myself to *choose* joy and happiness. I didn't feel happy at all, but as time passed it became a little easier to get out of bed in the morning.

One Sunday, James and I visited a new church. It was our first Sunday at Crossline Community Church. The pastor spoke on miracles, and he taught that this was a church that believed in miracles and was going to be praying for miracles in the lives of the people in this church and in this community.

James and I went home, and we decided that we were going to pray for miracles.

We decided that the only hope we had was to pray and ask God to heal our broken hearts and to heal our baby girl Kiley Joy.

We sent out 500 letters to family and friends, telling Kiley Joy's story. In the letter we included a fridge magnet with a picture of Kiley Joy with a Bible verse underneath that said, "The things Impossible with men, are possible with Christ" (Luke 18:27). The letter was an invitation to meet us on Tuesday nights at 7:00 p.m. to pray for miracles for our angel, Kiley Joy.

We met the following Tuesday at 7:00 p.m. Family and friends joined us, and we prayed for miracles in Kiley's life. We prayed that God would heal her. We prayed that this little girl would walk and talk.

Six years later, we continue to pray for miracles every Tuesday night at 7:00 p.m. Some nights there have been over forty people in attendance to pray over her, and some nights it is a quiet group of three or more. People from all over the world have prayed for miracles in Kiley Joy's life! Her story has been told on the radio. A missionary team from China blessed us with their prayers one Tuesday night when they were here in the states. We often enter homes where her fridge magnet still hangs after six years as a small reminder to pray for miracles!

It has been 300 plus Tuesday nights, praying for miracles, praying against the statistics.

So when we come together on a Tuesday night, we are confident that we have an army of prayer warriors around the world praying for miracles in her little life.

We believe that faith and prayers move God to action. We believe that "the things impossible with men are possible with Christ" (Luke 18:27).

We have faith in Jesus Christ and the hope for a miracle that allows us to choose joy and happiness each new day!

In early September 2008, our church prayed for Kiley Joy during a service focused on prayer and God and His power and promise of miracles.

One week later, at the age of four years old, our sweet angel Kiley Joy took her first steps. It has been an amazing miracle to see her develop, to walk, and to run!

We are excited to see what God is going to do next. We will pray everyday for a miracle! And, while we wait for our miracle, we *choose* joy.

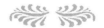

PRAYERS FOR KILEY JOY

By Kiley Joy's friends and family,
who have been praying for miracles every Tuesday night,
at 7 p.m. for the past six years.

Kiley Joy, you bring so much joy to our life in your own unique way: your smile, contagious laugh, sparkling blue eyes, and your love for people. Your life has taught us to love deeply, believe whole-heartedly, and pray boldly. We don't know anyone that has had so great an impact in only five years of life without saying a word. You are heard through your love for life.

Luke 18:27 "What is impossible with men, is possible with God."

Praying for miracles! We love you so…

—Mommy and Daddy
(Gini and James Williams)

NICKNAMES

Kiley Joy Williams. This is the name of the firstborn daughter of Gini and James Williams. Kiley Joy has Angelman syndrome. This however, does not tell us who she is. Kiley Joy has been given many nicknames, all of which are inspired by who Kiley is to us.

Kiley My Joy—Kiley brings such joy to our lives. She brings such great delight and happiness by her laughter, her quiet and gentle spirit, and her sweet heart. She will follow you around the house, because she loves to be near you. She loves people, and people love her, because there is something so wonderful about her that you cannot put into words. Joy spills from her life and into the lives of all who know her.

Pretty—Kiley Joy truly is one of the prettiest little girls you have ever seen: sparkling blue eyes that glint with joy when you walk in the door. Her hair is as golden as the sunshine. Her smile, well, her smile inspires. No matter how down, angry, tired, or depressed you may be, when you see her smile, you just have to smile back. Kiley Joy radiates, and everyday she lives up to the nickname *Pretty*.

The Flash—Man, oh, man is Kiley fast. Like a flash of lightening, she is getting into the grapes, your lunch, the paint, the...oh no! Who left the bathroom door open! Who knew that a child like Kiley had superhuman powers to get across the room and into a mess before you could even blink.

Poop Licker —This is the name given after the multiple instances when the unpleasing aroma of poopies hits as you walk into her room. Just when you think that you are going to greet a precious child with sleep in her eyes and a smile on her face, you, instead, realize that she has been into her poopie diaper and has proceeded to finger paint the walls, crib, even her own body with what seems to be an inhuman amount of poop. Those are the fun mornings where a bath and washing the crib sheets is guaranteed.

Frankenstein—One of the most inspiring sights I have ever seen was Kiley Joy walking. With her hands out in front, her feet a little unsure, she sways and swaggers as she makes her way across the room. When so many of the stories tell us she might never be able to walk, this child has overcome. Our little Frankenstein can walk and what a sight it is.

Destructor —There is no such thing as a clean room with Kiley around. What was once ordered and organized will soon become chaos in a matter of moments with Kiley. Pick up the balls? Why bother. Hide the blocks? She will find them. Store the videos in the cabinet? They have become boxes of art arranged in no particular pattern all over the floor. Kiley has refined this talent of destruction to make it an art form, and you can never get upset, because each mess is finished with the most innocent of smiles that makes it all okay.

Ki-Ki—This is the quickie, the one name that gets a smile every time. It is the name of affection that we call our girl. She is our *Ki-Ki*, a precious girl that brings so much to our lives.

I love Kiley Joy. She holds a special and very dear place in my heart. Her name, Kiley Joy, especially when spoken in prayer, inspires hope for the future, excitement for the things God has in store, and for the miracles He will work.

—Vanessa

MEMORIES

One Tuesday evening I came to prayer for Kiley. For a myriad of reasons I was feeling low. A fog was hanging over me, a familiar fog that has found its way into my life many, many times. Earlier that day a friend had just shared with me a wonderful verse from Isaiah 61 that says, "He has sent one filled with the Spirit to bring a garment of praise instead of a spirit of despair." As I sat in that classroom, listening to all the beautiful prayers for Kiley, I was stuck in my own fog, feeling the spirit of despair. All of a sudden little Kiley crawls over to me, pulls herself up by my knee, and looks into my face and smiles that wonderful smile at me. At that moment

I realized that Kiley was the one filled with the Spirit bringing to me a garment of praise. All I had to do was trade the garment of despair for the sweet love of God I saw in Kiley's eyes and on her face. Instantly I was so filled with joy, praise instead of despair. Kiley is filled with a spirit that is so right for this world. I can praise God for making Kiley and for the miracle He is doing through her to make us all a bit more like Him!

—John

My favorite time with Kiley Joy is when, for whatever reason, I am chosen to be the recipient of the *most* amazing snuggles and hugs I have ever known. When she was younger, she would come to me crawling and smiling, with little or no sound. Now, she comes toward me, walking with arms outstretched, smiling, and cooing, and laughing! She wraps her arms around my neck, lays her head on my shoulder, and the entire world is right. Kiley gets such a kick out of other children. My son, Cole, adores Kiley. I love the smile on his face when she toddles toward him, grabs his head, and looks right at him, laughing and making joyful sounds (that he is sure are words!). The depth of emotion, hope, and compassion that she brings out in him, as well as everyone else around her, is priceless. I have seen God's work in you and my faith has grown because of you.

We love you sweet girl!

—Nori and Cole

I was running around, doing errands in my car with all four of my kids plus Kiley Joy and her sister, Addison. My boys started fighting, Addison was screaming, Kenna was crying, and I was about to join her when I looked in my rearview mirror, and there was Kiley, smiling and giggling at me. I suddenly felt like I could handle all the chaos. When I walk in a room and see Kiley, the smile she gives me makes me feel like I am the most important person in the world. When she wraps her arms around me and hugs me, I could stay there all day. I just wish she would smile. There was a day when my precious sister Gini (mother to Kiley), sat crying as her heart was breaking, because Kiley would not be able to run and laugh with her cousins. But, just the other day I sat and smiled and thanked the Lord as I watched Kiley run and play with her cousins. Thank God for big and little miracles. The innocence and joy I see in Kiley Joy keeps things in perspective. Oh, if we all could see life through her eyes. I love you sweet Kiley

—Aunt Lisa

Everyone was busy at Grandma and Grandpa William's home for Addison's first birthday. Kiley Joy was watching all the excitement. I joined her outside and she took my hands. We walked all the way around the backyard, through the house, and back outside again. She worked so desperately to make each step and smiled continually as we walked. I was so proud of her and thrilled to think we had taken that very long walk together.

Each time we met after that it seemed she wanted to go walking with Aunt Gail, which tickled me to pieces. I wanted her to be able to do it all by herself and knew with her determination she would. She was going up and down the stairs, holding on and later walking around anything she could hold on too. She still had not made the journey independently. I kept thinking and praying she would. As I began a new school year, I shared with the kids in my kindergarten class my desire that she would be able to walk. Their family decided to start praying that she would walk before she was four. It was the beginning of school, and her birthday was in September. I did not know that Kiley Joy was trying really hard and had almost mastered the skill. Then just before her birthday she came to visit me. She started to reach out to me, and I was afraid she would fall, but to my delight, she walked over to me, and I got the best hug ever. Now just a couple months later I played with her on the jungle gym at school. She climbed, she smiled, she laughed, and, more than anything else, she shared that moment in time with me. The kids saw her walk to them and tried to join their line. They kept saying, "Look Mrs. Newton, Kiley is walking with us." Yes, she's walking and once again the prayers of children showed us that all things are possible with God. I love my Kiley Joy.

—Aunt Gail

Every time I see Kiley she lights up my day. She always greets me with a big smile and wanting a hug.

One of my fondest memories was just after she started to walk. I picked her up at the back of the church, and she wanted to walk all the way out. As she looked around and was walking with the crowd you could tell she was very proud of herself, and I was too. She had become a big girl.

—Grandpa (aka Pukka)

This old great-grandmom was so thrilled when you were born. You were such a beautiful baby. You stole my heart at first sight. None of your big, loving family could take their eyes off of you.

I remember your first smiles. Then your second Christmas, in your beautiful dress, you showed us you could move on your stomach and toes. Soon you were on your knees and crawling. What a thrill! Then you could climb on top of everything. The most amazing thing I watched you do was get on the piano bench. Then you were standing on the keys, trying to reach something on top of the piano. After many prayers, you walked before you were four. Now you are in school. What an amazing little girl!

I have loved the smiles on your face when any of the family comes in the room. It is so much fun to watch you wrestle with your dad and grandad. You just love rough play and tickles. The smiles turn to loud giggles.

When I see you I think you are a beautiful little angel. I am so lucky to have lived long enough to enjoy you, Addison and Grace.

I'll be watching you for more antics. You are so dear to me.

I love you.

—Great Grandmom

SOURCE OF JOY

Our Kiley Joy:

- is a source of joy to all who meet her

- is a symbol of hope

- - is living and breathing proof that God hears our prayers

- is a reminder that a medical diagnosis brings man's words, but God has the last word

- makes us look forward to heaven where all things are healed and made whole

- helps us understand the calling and privilege from God to parents of special needs children

- there is no one else like her, she is our treasure

- helps us love God more as we see him answer our prayers

- is a reward and our lives our richer because of her

- With love from me to you.

—Reenie

PRAYERS FROM COUSINS

- I am thankful that she walks, and I love to wrestle her. Kashton (four years old)

- I love Kiley. I see a happy face when I see her. Kenna (three years old)

- I Love Kiley's beautiful smile. I am praying that God gives her words. Cade (ten years old)

- Dear Lord, please help Kiley to skip. Amen, Chase (his bedtime prayer).

AUDREY LOUISE BEEGHLY

Elizabeth is a someone her daughter should hold in very high regard, as she is the toughest advocate I have ever had the pleasure to meet. I love the honesty of her story.

PLAYING ON THE OUTSIDE

By Elizabeth Beeghly
Mother to Audrey

Audrey, at age three, entered preschool in the fall of 2008. Early Intervention (EI) preschool, our natural first choice, underwhelmed us and overwhelmed Audrey. In Portland, OR, the EI system is broken. In a classroom, there are sixteen kids, a teacher, and two aides. Eight of the kids are special needs (all with different levels of functioning and needs), and the other eight are typical peers. No controls are placed on sex, need, or functioning level.

From the first day, Audrey seemed lost and unhappy. When Audrey started to become anxious—when we left the house to go to school and when we arrived—she was clearly telling me no, and so I pulled her from the school.

Around the same time, a local family preschool contacted Audrey about joining their community. It's a random lottery to secure a spot, so we were lucky. I walked into the school and got a good feeling about the program. Teacher Susan was kind, caring, soft-spoken, and wanted to learn about Audrey. At the first class, she introduced Audrey to the community and went over way to play with her and make her feel welcome. Because it is a free form school, there are no expectations. Just do what you like. Audrey is good at that. She attends the school with her respite care provider, Shelli (1:1 aide).

After several months some of the children started to engage Audrey in the classroom. Still, she is having some challenges in this environment. From the noise of the classroom frightening her to confusions about trying to keep up with her peers, each day is filled with challenges. I am confident that this is the best environment for Audrey to take steps toward the world of school.

It's hard to watch Audrey always playing on the outside. She drools, is clumsy, smiles too big, screams, puts her fingers in her mouth, sucks on things, gets into peoples personal space, and wants to play. Kids and parents alike are awkward and stand offish around her. Some kids even run away, flinch, or seem repulsed by her approach. When this happens, Audrey gets frustrated and begins to hit, kick, push, swing, throw things, etc. I think she is just trying to say what's wrong with me. Sometimes I've witnessed a child reject her, and she will throw herself to the ground and bang her head. Clearly this rejection hurts her feelings.

I find myself trying to befriend all of these children for Audrey. I learn their names, help to facilitate play, talk with their mothers—saying she is okay and wants to be your child's friend. Still we have no play dates, no birthday party invites, and no friends her age that get excited when they see her.

For Audrey and I, one of the most challenging aspects of our relationship is understanding and being understood. Since we spend every day together (I can count the number of days I have been away from her for more than a couple of hours on one hand), we understand each other on the basics: hungry and thirsty. The rest of our communication falls into a gray area.

Since infancy, I've worked hard at communication with my daughter. While exploring communication techniques, we have tried picture exchange, sign language, and ABS therapy. The next step will be a communication device. Audrey understands English pretty well. She's very lucky to have a mother and a sister who love to be demonstrative with our movements and speech. She can follow instructions that are directed at her and even follow conversations that are happening around her. More than once she has surprised me by starting to cry after telling her dad that I am going to the store.

Audrey is very good at picking up cues that tell her what is going on. For example, when the respite provider comes, that means mom is leaving; when her sister puts her jacket on, that means sister is leaving; when mom turns on the shower, it is time for Audrey to get naked. Audrey is always paying attention to what is happening around her.

UNDERSTANDING AUDREY

For me, understanding Audrey is a skill that I'm working on perfecting. It means spending lots of time with her each day, noticing precursors, surrounding and connecting the blurry dots to understand how she is feeling, and whatever her needs might be. I know there are numerous head, arm, and leg movements, as well as vocalizations, that are connected to specific things she is trying to communicate.

Most people understand her meaning when she shakes her head no and when she points to an item that means, "I want that." Crying means something is wrong, but it is sometimes impossible to know what is wrong. Audrey clearly has things to say. Even though I am tuned in to feelings and emotions, it is still a struggle to understand everything she is trying to say.

Audrey started physical, occupational, and feeding therapy at ten months of age. This was a busy time for our family, running from therapy to therapy as well as trying to work on all the techniques at home. It soon became overwhelming, and now we attend one combined therapy: Occupational-Sensory Integration and Speech. We also receive one weekly visit from a teacher from EI to work with Audrey on the STAR program. Six times per week, a respite care provider comes out to our home to work with Audrey (getting her used to people outside of our immediate family). They take her on social outings like the library, playground, and swimming pool among others. In my opinion, these are the most beneficial therapies.

PRETENDING

One week I spent some time with moms raising typical children. The first event was Audrey's cooperative pre-school's monthly membership meeting, and the second was at Madeleine's (our other daughter), fifth birthday party.

I find it hard to be happy at these events, meeting other parents and children for the first time; pretending that my life is great, that I am just like them. Not wanting anyone to know the truth, that Audrey had seizures all day and all night for the past two weeks, and that I am starting to see regression, or that Audrey is drooling and seems off-balance. I don's want to scare people off too soon. I want to have things in common first before I let them dive in to my foreign world of disability and an unhealthy child.

At the cooperative preschool meeting, we played a game and then discussed how we thought our children would play. I had no idea what to say. My daughter doesn't play games except peek-a-boo. She hides, and we find her. Do I tell the other parents and have the ensuing awkward silence reveal how different our experiences are? Do I tell them the truth or just compare Madeleine to their children? My mind works. I don't know what to say. I wish for the meeting to be over so I can get home. A poor soul comes over to check on me, and I tell her what I am feeling. She says that she is sorry and that she had not clue and walks away.

A few days later it was Madeleine's fifth birthday party. It was held at a local indoor pool. Shelli, our respite care provider, accompanied us to keep an eye on Audrey and to enable Brian (my husband), and I to focus our attention on the birthday girl and her guests. It was a mixture of pleasure and pain as I watched Audrey smiling so uninhibitedly at everyone. She had started to get over her stranger anxiety. I found myself watching the other parents check her out and watch as they figured out that something wasn't right. How their expressions changed. Did I see pity? It bothered me, right or wrong. Thank goodness I was too busy to watch.

For the first three years of Audrey's life it wasn't obvious to most people that she wasn't like everyone else. Her disability was hidden. Now I do not have the luxury of people looking past what is right in front of their face. People see her. They see me struggling to keep up with her. In less than one minute, she could hit me, bite me, smile at me, have a seizure, cry, and try to run away. This is it. This is my reality.

It is hard for some people to handle. It is hard for me to handle. I am learning. I will help other parents understand. I will have friends again, someday.

AVA CARLASSARE

Profound is the only word I can come up with to describe this, one of my favorite submissions. I think you will agree.

ENTERING OZ

By Andrea Carlassare
Mother to Ava

Leaving the doctor's office, I felt like I had been punched in the stomach. I didn't think I would be able to find the car in the parking garage. I had been confident that the evaluation by the developmental pediatrician would tell me that all of my daughter's issues—her motor delays, lack of speech, and excessive reflux—were all due to low muscle tone and not to worry. I had assumed that the lack of growth in her head circumference that had become evident at her last well-baby visit had been the result of human error and nothing else. But, instead, after a thorough evaluation of my daughter, the doctor told me that the delays were *significant* and that genetic tests should be run. The shock hit me as I entered the elevator to leave the building. The drive home was a blur.

I searched for all the support and reassurance I could find on that first evening. My mother consoled me with the analogy from the *Welcome to Holland* essay by Emily Perl Kingsley. In the essay, the experience of raising a child with a disability is described as anticipating a trip to Italy, but instead finding oneself in Holland when the flight lands. Since that first night, many others have referenced the words in that essay.

Six months later and with a confirmed diagnosis of Angelman syndrome, I have reflected on my initial emotions. I am thankful that I am through the early adjustment phase. I feel myself regaining my balance in life and spirit. And I ponder the Kingsley essay each time I pass it, now posted on my fridge. I love the simplicity of the analogy and its ability to reassure, but my vision of arriving in Holland by airplane is too placid and not in concert with the emotions I felt. I searched for an analogy that better fit my frame of mind. I settled on the whirlwind arrival of Dorothy to the Land of Oz. Yes, arriving involuntarily by tornado, flattened to the ground in fear, instead of sipping cranberry juice inside an air conditioned airplane, seemed to be a much more applicable image.

The news I received that day completely upended me. It changed how I viewed myself, my future, my family, people with disabilities, and society. I felt like Dorothy in the tornado. I had been anticipating my return to the familiar comfort of home and its routines after the doctor's visit, when instead I was forced abruptly and unwillingly into another place. The familiar was spun around and turned upside down. I was left dizzy with the amount of raw emotions and thoughts swirling inside of me. But I had to swiftly make sense of the new place I had landed. I was in a new place and many of my possessions, carefully organized into my trunk labeled *Hopes, Dreams, and Expectations*, had been thrown out the window and shattered. I had to hurriedly pack an arsenal bag so I could begin to navigate my way through this new world. I had to quickly make sense of the diagnosis and the available therapies, social services, and community supports. I was now part of a club I had never anticipated belonging to; I had entered the subculture of the disabled. I had to discard the thoughts that would no longer be beneficial to me or to my daughter. I had to confront prejudices I held and start to quiet the unease I have toward people that are cognitively disabled. I had to do all of this and still function as a mother, wife, and friend. Dorothy's moment of shock passed in seconds as she entered and accepted the strangeness of Oz. My moment of shock reverberated for months.

I rejoined Dorothy as she walked the yellow, brick road, searching to find her home again. As I began to establish a new routine filled with doctors and therapists, I began to find a new daily rhythm. I met fabulous new friends that had already walked the path and were comfortable in this new world. Like the Tin Man, the Lion, and the Scarecrow, these friends all shared with me their hearts, their courage, and their knowledge. They continue to give me directions and guide me on this unfamiliar path. They keep me marching forward instead of slipping back.

Like the Wicked Witch's monkeys, chasing Dorothy, I walk with the shadow of fears dancing around me. *When will the seizures start? What will we happen to my daughter after my husband and I are dead? Will my family ever be able to go on a lengthy vacation again? How will my husband and I enjoy our retirement?* These fears pick at me. I am constantly pushing them away and redirecting my thoughts to the present day. If I keep the anxiety at bay and stay in the present moment. I give myself the emotional space to keep moving forward. I remind myself that there is no need to expend effort worrying about the future. No one knows what the future holds. My daughter's unexpected diagnosis drove home that point. We cannot anticipate or control what may happen in our lives. We can only make the best of what currently is. If the present moment is good, then I will enjoy it. If the present moment is difficult, then I will just remember to breath. If I enjoy my journey on the path today, and if I continue to walk a bit forward each day, then soon I will be able to look back and find that I have traveled far and that it has been on a bright and shining road.

When Dorothy returned home, she struggled to explain the wonders of Oz. I struggle to reconcile the absolute joy that my daughter brings me with the views that society holds on the disabled. Her diagnosis does not change who she is or reduce the amount of happiness she brings to me. The disability does not make my daughter less of a person; it does not make us less of a family. But it does change how she is seen by society. I wish I could make everyone understand that my daughter's challenges because of Angelman syndrome are just one part of her. Like any other human, she will make the best of the cards she has been dealt. We are all different from one another. *Different* is not a negative term, but a neutral one. A disability does not make us better or worse, just different.

Dorothy's memories of Oz gave her a better understanding and appreciation of her world. For myself, I have realized that what has changed is not my life, but my assumptions of what my life would hold for me in the future. My life is still the same as the day before we were told something was amiss with our daughter. She remains the same delightful little girl. Yes, my routines have changed, I have widened my circle of friends, I have expanded my views, and I have examined my strengths and weaknesses, but really I have just inched forward on this path that represents my life. It is still the same path I was on six months ago, the tornado just plopped me down around the next bend, and I got my breath taken away by the new view. I also may have hit a patch of ice and slipped a few times, but now I am up and trotting along again. And know that I realize that I am still on the same path—that there was only a change in scenery. I have also recognized that there is no need to yearn for home. I have awoken and realized that I am still there.

PATRICIA SCHIFFELERS

I met Christa Schiffelers, Lisa Veniza and Amy Boyd in Canada, at my first Angelman. I was very impressed with her attitude towards her daughter. She was so positive and told me that she never apologizes for her daughters' behavior. If she grabs someone's hand or takes something off someone's plate she just smiles. She and Trisha's awesome support staff were very interested in my book project and on the last day of the conference she approached me with a list of possible titles for the book that she along with her daughters' caregivers had come up with. Some of the titles included: 'These Our Special Angles', 'To Love an Angel', 'Angels Walking Amongst Us', 'Angel Tales' and 'Beautiful Angels'. Even though I did not use any of their titles for the book, their list was a catalyst to finding the perfect title to the book that we all share.

SOCIAL BUTTERFLY

By Christa Schiffelers
Mother to Patricia

My daughter, Patricia, was born thirty-two years ago, it took twenty-five years to diagnose her with Angelman syndrome.

When she was born she had some medical problems. At first we thought she had a heart condition, but it turned out her heart was fine. She was diagnosed at the age of four weeks with Androgen Insensitivity syndrome and at ten months old, a team of doctors, except for one, felt that she had cerebral palsy.

Patricia is in a wheelchair, cannot speak, and is severely disabled. At the age of eighteen we had to make the decision to have a feeding tube put in, as she would not eat or drink and lost a lot of weight.

When Patricia was twenty-five years old we asked her geneticist if he would do some genetic testing, as we never believed she had cerebral palsy, and we wanted to know what she had. He agreed to do the testing, and it turned out she had a very large deletion of the fifteenth chromosome and was diagnosed with Angelman syndrome. We were very relieved to have the proper diagnosis.

When Patricia was nineteen years old we set up a not-for-profit society for her, under the British Columbia Societies Act, and negotiated a contract. At that time it was set up with the Ministry of Health, now the society contracts with CLBC.

The same year she was diagnosed, we found out there was an Angelman Conference in Vancouver, BC. We were all very excited to attend and to have an opportunity to meet with other angels. Patricia, three of her support staff, and myself were able to go to this extraordinary event. Patricia's geneticist even did a whole session on Patricia.

We have learned a lot over the years about how to care for Patricia, but wish we had known a long time ago that she had Angelman syndrome. Patricia lives at home in her own suite, attached to our home. She has a wonderful team of support staff that care for her. My husband and I do the nightshifts. Now that my husband is retired we have a chance to get away on holidays and feel secure that Patricia is well looked after. We have been told many times that we are the lucky ones that get the honor of looking after her.

Patricia loves to participate in the community, and everyone around here knows her. When we are out in the community people come up to her to chat. We always give her heck that she does not introduce us, as they just talk away to her, and many times just ignore us. We always ask her, "Who was that?" and she just gives us a big smile and laughs!

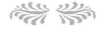

FASTEST ARMS IN THE WEST

By Lisa Vezina
Support Staff and friend to Patricia

I started working with Patricia four years ago. Her special smile, innocent blue eyes, and flaming red hair had me fooled for several months. It wasn't until she grabbed a hot dog from a poor, unsuspecting two-year-old girl and gobbled it down, laughing like a devil, that I discovered the real Patricia and knew what I was dealing with. She has the longest, fastest arms in the west and can swipe a cookie before you know it is gone. This is usually followed by hysterical laughter.

Although usually Patricia is happy and healthy, she does have her down times. The most frustrating thing for me is when she is not feeling well and hurting. She cannot tell me where it hurts, and she must wonder why we cannot take the pain away. This is the most difficult part about knowing an Angel.

Patricia has gotten to know me now, and she knows she has to work extra hard to pull one over on me, but she still manages to do this; must be the red hair.

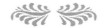

KIND OF A REBEL

By Amy Boyd
Ambassador for Patricia

This Angel came into my life in August 2006, but I feel like I have known her my whole life. She has an amazing love for life that I think we all can learn from. While we are all preoccupied with ourselves, she truly enjoys life. She has the highest sense of self-esteem of anyone I have ever met. She doesn't worry if her hair is in the right place, or if she is skinny enough, or if people will like her. She accepts people as they are and doesn't care what people think of her; she is who she is. Wouldn't life be great if we all could be like her?

Trisha has a great love for water and swimming, although the hot tub is her favorite part. I'm pretty sure it is the only reason she goes swimming. She loves music and is so spoiled that she has a million musical toys, and she knows how to work them better than I do. If I can't get one working I just hand it to her, and she has it going in a second. She loves it when you make funny noises. If you do, you're sure to get a big laugh.

Trish is kind of a rebel. If you say her name like she is in trouble, she gets so excited she doesn't know what to do with herself. She loves to chew, chew, chew, but I am sure that is no surprise to any of you who know any Angels. She has several great chewy toys that are in the shape of Ps and Qs, so mind your Ps and Qs everyone. She loves parties and thinks any event that is thrown is specifically for her; she thinks she is always the guest of honor. Presents are good, but she really just loves the paper and will spend hours making sure it is shredded in just the right way.

When she laughs you can hear what her voice would sound like if she could talk. Sometimes it sounds like she might just blurt something out. She hates to brush her teeth but loves to chew on the toothbrush. She loves to go to the movies and starts bouncing up and down when you are in the parking lot of the theater. She *loves* her bed. When getting her ready for bed at night, she is so happy, although she doesn't sleep much—go figure. She has a great love for the outdoors. If you sit her on the lawn she will pull the grass right out by the roots and cover herself in dirt, and all you can see are the whites of her eyes.

Trisha has unbelievable patience. While we can all get annoyed, waiting in a doctors office when the doctor is behind, you can be sure Trisha will have a big smile on her face and will keep everyone in the waiting room occupied with her laughter. Trisha has the most amazing hair; it is fiery red and super thick. I love doing her hair in the morning. She has great determination and, although she is nonverbal, she communicates her wants and desires quite clearly. There is not a day that goes by that I spend with her that she doesn't have me in stitches at some point during the day.

Patricia Schiffelers is loving, happy, determined, content, a good friend, a daughter, inspirational, caring, patient, beautiful, and confident. Although she is disabled she is perfect just the way she is, and we are better people for knowing her.

SAMUEL HICKEY

I thought I had received all the submissions I was going to receive so when I received this unexpected story from a brother to an Angel my heart leapt for joy! I absolutely love reading siblings versions of their experiences and insight into living with an Angel sibling. I want my boys to appreciate their brother and learn as much as Andy has from Samuel.

MY LIFE WITH SAMUEL
By Andy Hickey
Brother to Samuel

My brother, Sam, has Angelman syndrome. He can't walk or talk. He does possess an extremely happy demeanor. I'm not going to lie; living with Sam has definitely had its ups and downs.

Everyone's moments (and I'm sure you already have plenty), are going to be different than mine. I want to tell you what I have learned from Sam and why I feel blessed to have him for a brother. At my ripe old age of twenty, I am comfortable saying that I don't have everything figured out, but I do know a thing or two about growing up with a sibling who has special needs. I am going to share with you what Sam has taught me over the last fifteen years, and I hope that you can relate these ideas to your brother or sister. What I am going to discuss has helped me appreciate my brother more, and above all, appreciate life more. To be completely honest, I wouldn't be who I am if it wasn't for Sam. He has made my life better, and I hope that by the time you are twenty, you will feel the same way about your brother or sister. So sit back and get ready to soak it all in, because this is some good stuff.

The first and most beneficial thing you can do in your life is find out exactly what is wrong with your sibling. Ask your parents about their condition; if they don't know all that much, consult the Internet or a book. If it is a known disorder, there is information on it. Knowing what is scientifically wrong will help you understand situations better and more importantly understand them better. This information is invaluable and will make life a lot easier, trust me!

Now I am going to talk about the small things. Don't sweat the small things your sibling does. Sam was such a terror when he was younger. I could rant and rave about this all day, but I'm not going to put you through that. The main thing that I want you to understand is that these things happen. Something of yours is going to get broken and there really is nothing you can do about it. Your sibling is going to do things that infuriate you; feel free to get mad, it helps you feel better. It isn't good to bottle up your frustrations, because you'll probably end up doing something you'll regret. But remember, you can't hold a grudge against your brother or sister, because most of the things that happen are not only out of your control, but out of their control as well. I am absolutely positive that Sam would not do half of the things he does if he was physically capable of doing it the right way.

You need to be patient with your brother or sister. Physiologically speaking, they may be incapable of doing what you can do, and you have to realize this. There are going to be moments in your life where you have to show infinite patience, and you are going to have to be prepared for that. When you get frustrated with them, try putting yourself in their position and think about how you would want to be treated. You may think your life is rough, but I promise the ordeals they face on a day-to-day basis are exponentially worse.

Find things about your sibling that you appreciate. Sam was having his cognitive ability analyzed in San Diego, and the doctor was having him put a string of beads inside of a small cup that was shaped like a film canister. Sam was having a really hard time with it, because his movements are so jerky (the poor guy has big problems with fine motor skills). Instead of getting angry and giving up, he stayed very calm and methodically kept trying to put the string of beads in the cup. I can't remember if he actually got the beads into the cup, I just remember how patient and calm he was during the situation. Anytime I get frustrated when I am having a hard time doing something I think about how insistent and unrelenting, yet tranquil, Sam was when trying to put those beads in that cup. It's moments like this that you have to notice about your sibling and cherish, because they can teach you so much about the right way to approach life. I can honestly say that since that test I have been a calmer, more collected person, or at least have tried to be. If you take the time to appreciate the demeanor of your sibling during the moments of their struggle, you can and will find ways to better yourself.

Lastly, but most definitely not least, be proud of your sibling. Always refer to them as your brother or your sister with enthusiasm. When telling someone a story involving your sibling, don't make it a point to inform the person that they are disabled. But don't be afraid to talk with someone about your sibling's disability. Just as you wouldn't introduce your sibling as your "sister with a size six foot," you shouldn't introduce them as your "sister with Autism." This immediately applies an unnecessary label to your brother or sister. The person you are telling the story to will no longer see a person, they will see a disability. Let them hear your story before categorizing your sibling. I never think of my brother as my disabled brother, he is just my brother. I know he is disabled, but I never refer to him as being disabled. I tell people he has Angelman syndrome, but only after they have an idea of whom Sam the person is.

SEAN TUNBRIDGE

I relate to this story from Jane on so many levels. Not only the running, but learning to take each day at a time.

I WILL FIGHT IN HIS CORNER

By Jane Tunbridge
Mother to Sean

Looking at life through Sean's eyes, everything is perfect. We have leaned to take each day as it comes and not to worry about the silly little things. We have to be strong for him and our other children. We all accept that Sean is different and special.

We are very involved in Gibraltar, which is a close-knit community. Our family also helps out. At the beginning, it took my parents a while to understand the scientific side of Sean's diagnosis. But they love Sean and accept him for who he is and take him out as they would our other children.

When we received the diagnosis it painted a very bleak future for us. I would have been a very different person, had it not been for Sean. I used to be very shy and reserved; now I am a marathon woman! I do half-marathons, help out at his school, and I talk to doctors as if I know more than they do! I will fight in Sean's corner with whomever I have to, to get the results that I want.

On really bad days I cry a bit, then I pick myself up, brush it off, go for a run, or do something fun with Sean, if I have the energy.

ABIGAIL GEORGE

This story about Abby gave me such joy as I read how her older siblings argued over who had helped to teach her what first.

I'M THE MAN

By Susan George
Mother to Abby

The memories of Abby's accomplishments bring me a lot of joy, especially the talking ones. She started saying occasional words and phrases that really surprised us when she was between two-and-a-half and three years old. Most of the things she said we only heard once or twice. She started to say, "Mama," to me. She would say it all day long, but I didn't mind! The longest things she has said are, "Robby I love you," "Nana Joan," and "I'm the man." The latter phrase was influenced by her older brother!

Although she doesn't converse or ask for what she wants, she often comes out with funny things like, "Aflac," while watching TV. She has sung her own mumbled version of the first few measures of the Hannah Montana theme song, amazingly in tune, until she got sick of the show. The things we hear on a more daily basis are, "Mama," "Papa," and "Brabra."

It was she who decided that *Papa* is easier to say than *Dada*, but she also says it to her pop-pop. She has only said, "Father," twice. "Brabra," is *brother*, which she affectionately calls her brothers and sister. It makes me happy that she is able to vocally acknowledge her siblings, as I know they play a greater role in her development than we ever imagined.

Her older sister worked very hard getting her to walk when she used to need a walker. Her older brother is always protecting her. Both of them argue who taught what first. Now that she is five years old, her three-year-old brother insists on taking her hand to lead her on walks when we go outside, and he is quick to report when she's in danger.

ELIJAH MICHAEL JAMES HUMPHRIES

I know that you will love this story as much as I do. It was one of the last stories that I received. I can't count how many times I have read and reread the tender words of an adoring father.

FAITH JOURNEY

By Darren Humphries
Father to Elijah

One of my most memorable experiences with my son, Elijah, was the Saturday mornings that I took him swimming after dropping off my wife and daughter at piano lessons. We drive across town for him to go swimming in a small pool with staff that was trained to work with children with disabilities. In the water, Elijah was in his element. In the swimming pool, Elijah could stand with the support of a foam ring and could walk. He was always sad when it was time to get out. One fun thing was trying to keep him in his car seat. One morning I was driving in our new car to the swimming pool, when I heard a funny noise. I turned to see that he had managed to open his passenger door. I pulled the car over and quickly engaged the child lock to stop that from occurring again.

The scariest moments of our life with Elijah both relate to seizures. When Elijah first started having seizures it was pretty dramatic; he would have as many as 150-200 drop seizures in one day. I knew that having seizures was likely to happen to Elijah, but nothing prepared me for having to watch as seizures took control of my son's body and feeling completely helpless.

The last seizures that Elijah had did not stop and resulted in massive brain damage and irreversible damage to his internal organs and muscle tissue. These were the seizures that would take his life. We realized once Elijah began having seizures that this would be something that would require treatment over a period of time. Never in my wildest dreams did I ever imagine that they would take his life. There were times during his hospital stay that left my wife, our daughter, and me emotionally rung out. We were devastated to learn the full extent of the damage to Elijah's body and that our dear son would not live.

We gathered our family and close friends to say goodbye, and then his life support was switched off, and he gently and quietly went on to eternal life in my arms. The journey since has been filled with grief and pain, but Elijah and his journey still continue to speak to many people. It is with the hope that we will be reunited with Elijah that keeps us on this journey of faith.

One of the most memorable and precious experiences I have is when my daughter, Francesca, painted Elijah's feet and made prints of them on paper. During the last day of Elijah's life, the nurse who cared for Elijah in the ICU suggested that Francesca might like to paint Elijah's hands and feet with poster paint and then take prints of them. This is one of the only times that Elijah would have been still enough for this to take place. Francesca lovingly painted Elijah's feet and hands and made prints of them on paper. Francesca has always dearly loved her brother and was excited to do this with him. The biggest thing she misses about her brother is play wrestling with him on the floor each day after school.

When Elijah was diagnosed with Angelman syndrome it was a great relief and a time of grief for us. One of the things that Elijah and Angelman syndrome have done for us is strengthen our family. We learned to slow down and celebrate the small things that Elijah learned to do, and these became more significant. Elijah crawled for so long, and we really celebrated when he pulled himself up. Elijah's Angelman syndrome led us to grow in areas of our faith journey for inner and personal strength for the journey ahead.

CEDRIC COBURN

The practice of separating people into boxes, lending us understanding to a certain event or 'type' of person, is comfortable and a common practice for many of us. What I love about this story is that when given a certain box by our circumstances or by others, we do not need to stay there unchanging: as we grow and learn, the box stretches.

THE BOX

By Samantha Coburn
Mother to Cedric

As humans we try to find the place where we fit—our box, the area that defines us to ourselves and to the communities around us. When we have our children we begin the process for them. It is natural. "I want Beth to grow up like so and so," "I hope David likes to do such and such," then our children start to create their own boxes with likes, dislikes, friends, and activities.

Sometimes our kiddos are given a box from birth: a genetic disorder, cerebral palsy, autism, the list goes on. As a parent we try to gain an understanding of this box. Sometimes the box is cerebral palsy, only to find out later it is really Angelman syndrome.

The change in diagnosis gave us a sense of relief; I know that may sound weird but, I had carried a huge amount of guilt over my son's birth. It wasn't easy, there was meconium. He had heart decelerations, because the cord was wrapped and crimped around his neck. The doctor had been inducing me for over a week, and I was exhausted.

I had talked to my doctor about doing a c-section but I wasn't very adamant about it. In hindsight I wish I had been. I ended up with an emergency c-section anyway. That hesitation has haunted me ever since. I wondered if things would have been different if I had stood up for my kiddo and myself; because of my weakness, did my kiddo suffer? So upon learning my son had Angelman syndrome that guilt was released. I had worked on releasing it for five years, but the diagnosis finally let me release it. I had been doing what needed to be done for my kiddo within my box of guilt, somehow trying to make up for what I believed were my deficiencies. Now there is a new box on our doorstep—Angelman syndrome.

What are the parameters of this box? Well there are general parameters in looking at the clinical diagnosis of what Angels can and cannot do. However it is through experience that I have found and been reminded that boxes stretch! It can be frustrating when it comes to services and schooling for special needs kiddos. We need a diagnosis—that box that says, "Oh yes you can get such and such," or, "No, you can't have such and such." Then once we have people and services in place, the battle to pull our kiddos out of their box begins.

I have found this especially difficult in the school district. It is difficult to get them to see that our kiddos benefit from certain services, maybe their progress isn't their idea of what it should be, but whether your kiddos progress as high as Mt. Everest or as low as a rolling hillside, the point is there is progress! My kiddos progress is a little like *The Little Engine that Could*, slowly moving up the hill, but he is moving and should it flatten out for a while, I know there is another slope on the way.

So my roar to myself and to all families out there is:

> Yes there is this box that gets hard to carry, that is ready to define limits on our kiddos from the outside world. *But...* this box stretches as our Angels light up our life everyday. Punch out those borders! Specialists may say one thing, but parents of special need kiddos, who are with their kiddos twenty-four seven in the trenches, know their kiddos best. Boxes are our guidelines but not our definition.

> We all know coloring and venturing out of those lines is where the joy of life begins!

There are times when words are caught in our bodies, stagnant and causing ill effects on our manner and mien. There are times when those words then flow and become wonderful healing opportunities for us. It is my hope that this bit of poetry is helpful to others as well. Enjoy...

A blessing was born upon a day
Near perfection in every way
Gathered in my arms you sleep
Ever full my heart, sadly it will weep
Lurking deep within your form
Missing pieces, will become the norm
Although my heart will roar
Nothing will heal this sore

Specialists line up in a row
Years fly by 'ere we find our foe
Now the answer is clear
Darling child, you're an angel dear
Rendered voiceless though you are
Opulent your soul shines like a star
My lamb, how blessed are we
Each moment with you, our beautiful destiny

JOSEPH HILL

One of our Early Intervention teachers asked us if we would be okay with giving out our contact information to other parents of Angelman children. The happy result was getting to meet Jennifer and Joseph. Jennifer has such a great attitude towards her life, and you get that feeling from reading her words.

FAMILY MEMORIES

By Jennifer Hill
Mother to Joseph

Some of our favorite family memories with Joseph have been during the Christmas holidays. On Joseph's second Christmas we found him cuddled under the tree with the presents and one of his sister's dolls. For his third Christmas, we were determined to find an appropriate riding toy that he could actually fit on and ride. We took him to the toy store and had him sit on various cars and trikes. We finally found a Radio Flyer tricycle with a belt and a sunroof that was just his size. When we attempted to remove Joseph from the tricycle, he screamed and threw a fit, so we knew that was the one! He had never behaved so badly in a store before. When we brought out the tricycle on Christmas morning, his face lit up.

One Christmas evening our other children had put out cookies for Santa only to see Joseph running down the hall, eating the cookies a moment later. He no doubt thought how cool it was that someone had left out some cookies for him!

With life being crazy and challenging at times, it is wonderful that we can look into Joseph's little face and see what a pure joy he really is.

When Joe was being evaluated for Early Intervention, two professional evaluators came to our home. One talked with me while the other (a psychologist), one was going to *play* with Joe and see where he was at developmentally. Once the psychologist was sitting on the floor, Joe decided it was *wrestle* time. Joe tackled the poor woman to the floor. Luckily our older son, Nolan—who was nine at the time—was there to rescue her, by pulling Joe off of her back and holding him. While he held Joe, she asked Nolan questions about Joe. The report we received from the evaluation was full of quotations from Nolan and notes from the psychologist agreeing with conclusions by our nine-year-old son!

Joseph likes to run around the house, *exploring*. By *exploring*, I mean "get into things." It is both frustrating and down right hilarious when he gets into something and then holds the item high in the air with a huge grin that seems to say, "Look what I got!" or, "I did it!" He just recently figured out how to turn on and off light switches. He runs around the house, giggling as he turns on one light and then turns another one off. It is the same grin as before, but this time it seems to be saying, "Look what I can do!"

If you sit down, Joseph assumes that you are his chair. He loves to cuddle, but he also loves to wrestle. So he may climb up on you to cuddle, or he may try to grab you to wrestle. He decides these things as the mood strikes him.

Joseph loves music, so much that when he hears it, he will run to the source. He will then come to a dead stop and listen for a moment, and then he will start swaying his upper body like a little dance. Joseph loves TV. He wants it on and on his show. He loves Sprout TV and anything with Elmo. He will tolerate cartoons and Disney and shows that his sister watches, but a football or basketball game? That is boring. He has been known to whack his daddy in the back of the head if a football game is on. Also, he changes the channel on the TV, which of course goes to static, and then he laughs. His other trick is to slap or push the TV in order to make his show come on. When that doesn't work he will push the TV over and look at you like, "What? It was on the wrong channel anyway."

Joseph is very, very, very social. If he gets to go to his brothers' or sisters' basketball or soccer games, he wants to run around and say hello (reach out his hand), to everyone there. He may not have the balance to get to all the places where people are sitting or standing, but he will not give up, and he finds a way to say hello. This of course makes it impossible to watch the game.

Joseph also loves to play hide and seek. His older siblings and their friends enjoy playing with him. Joseph is very good at finding people.

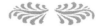

Jennifer has encapsulated Josephs' internal monologue so perfectly that I can't help but wonder if he didn't help her write this!

LIFE FROM JOSEPH'S POINT OF VIEW

Mom's van is cool. In Mom's van I get to go places. If my mom says, "Let's go for a ride," I am ready. I sit down by the front door to get my jacket and shoes on and then jump up and down until I am in the van. Then I laugh a happy laugh. Mom's van is cool.

The school bus comes too early. I do not want to get up. I do not want to eat. But I will eat my banana. I do not want to get on the bus. Hey! There is the neat bus driver lady! She might need a hug today. There are my friends. We are riding to school. Hey! There are my wonderful teachers! School is fun!

Elmo is cool. Binkies are cool. I don't care what you say, binkies are cool. I will stand up, put my arms back, move back and forth, and say, "Uuuuuraaa!" if you take my binky.

But plastic is the coolest. Ziploc sandwich bags are the coolest things ever. If you do not give me that plastic bag, I will grab it. If you still do not give me that bag, you are really going to hear me say, "Uuurrraaa!"

Baths are fun. I like running water. I will turn the faucet back on if you turn it off. I like to lie down in the bath. No, you better not turn off that water. I will splash! I splashed! That was funny. Oh, now they are making me get out of the bath. Still that was pretty funny. Man, what a good laugh. Oh, well I am dressed now. I wonder if Elmo is on. Nope, Lauren is watching *Hanna Montana*, but Nolan is doing homework. I can mess with Nolan! Nolan is not letting me get his homework. Oh well… big sigh… I will go and cuddle with Lauren and watch *Hanna Montana*. Hey, what is in that cabinet? I bet I can break that childproof lock. I think that is where the pans are. Hey that would be fun. Oh no. I am in time out. Still that was pretty funny even if I did not get in there. What a good laugh. Hey I can see the TV from here, and it is on my show!

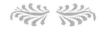

MY BROTHER

By Lauren Hill
Sister to Joseph

My brother is many different things. But one thing I never understood was why people said that they were sorry about him having Angelman syndrome, because I love him the way he is. So there is no need for people to say sorry.

CONRAD

Margie (who is my husband's Mother) has captured the spirit of Conrad and so many other Angels. If only we could know what our children know, really see what they see, I know we would all be better people.

CONRAD, THE PROFESSOR

By Margie Hunt
Grandmother to Conrad

Oh, if I could just be Conrad, if only for a day. To know what he knows, understand what he understands, feel the joy he shares with our Heavenly Father through a veil that must be much thinner for him than for the rest of us. Does he remember more of heaven than we do? Does he pray in ways we can't comprehend? Does he know he is here as a gift to us all? Will he teach us what he knows?

I remember when I first sensed that my beautiful, blond, blue-eyed, new grandson—the third of what would end up being a troupe of ten grandsons—might have developmental conditions. I was certain my son and daughter-in-law were concerned and beginning to seek professional advice. I carefully asked questions and waited. When my son, Matt, and daughter-in-law, Pam, shared the news with us of Conrad's diagnosis, I felt at first a sadness that was quickly replaced with an unexpected sense of elation. I knew this child would change their lives and would have hoped that they might not have such a challenge. But I also knew that Conrad would be a blessing in ways that we would all only begin to understand and appreciate over time. Life works in that way: those occurrences that seem like such a sacrifice in the beginning turn out to be blessings.

I recognize this was much easier for me to say. It would be Matt and Pam who would bear the greater burden—and receive the greater blessings—as the parents of a special needs child. They would experience the fear, anguish, uncertainty, and ongoing stress associated with Conrad's growth and development. They would learn a whole new way to parent, a whole new mode of child behaviors, and a whole new way to build and bond a family. They would learn to treat this child *special*, while never diminishing the same *specialness* in their other three sons. And they would learn to love and be loved by Conrad in the ways most meaningful to him.

Watching Matthew and Pamela as they raise Conrad is a privilege. It seems that Conrad brought with him the very characteristics his family would need in order to nurture him: patience, perseverance, courage, love, and kindness—all traits that are deeply ingrained in Conrad and, now, in the family DNA.

Conrad is, in fact, quite the professor, teaching all of us ever since he was born.

Conrad teaches me conviction. He doesn't just walk into a room, he owns it. He quickly scopes the scene, finds those things he most likes—magazines, books, candy, bathtubs, and a good cartoon show—and then gravitates to those individuals who give him the very best hugs…which he readily returns. Nothing's better than a Conrad two-armed hug. I love his hugs.

Conrad teaches me patient communication. He can't express his thoughts to me with words, but if I patiently wait and listen, truly listen, I can speak and hear his language, the sounds he utters and the sounds he does not. I love his speech.

Conrad teaches me joy. He laughs, not a little, like most Angelman children, but a lot and often. It's impossible not to laugh with him and, somehow, in the process, I feel more joyful and see the world a little more like he does. I love his laughter.

Conrad teaches me love. His heart is in his eyes. Sometimes, when he looks intensely in my eyes, I sense that he knows me very well—my faults, my weaknesses—and loves me in spite of them. I love his iridescent, approving eyes.

And Conrad teaches me faith. He is, without questions, a blessed gift to our family, one that could only have come from a loving Father in heaven.

Wiser than us all, Conrad continues to teach me every day. And if I'm not paying attention, he'll find the right time to look me straight in the eye. "Listen up, Grandma," I seem to hear him say, "be more patient, be more kind, be more understanding, be more tolerant, be who you're supposed to be. You can do it. I'll help you.

For many years, I have played a verbal game with my grandsons, asking them, "Who's the best boy?" To which they respond, "I am."

And then, I ask, "And do you know why I love you?" To which they respond, "Because I'm me!"

Conrad, you're the best boy… the best teacher, the best friend. And I thank the heavens every day that you're you.

PHOTOS

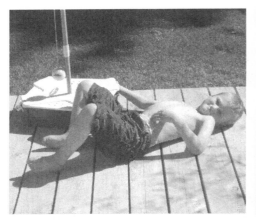

Connie in the backyard.

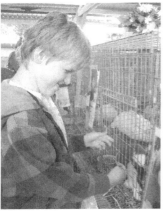

Connie at the county fair.

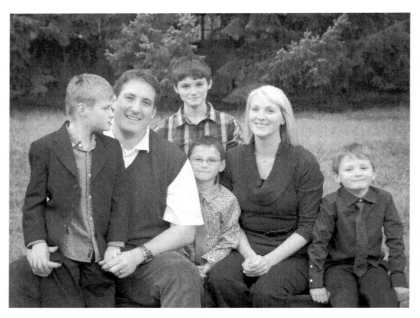

Family Picture 2011 (l-r) Conrad, Matt, Ben, Wilson, Pam, George

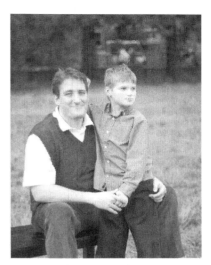

Conrad with his favorite
person - Matt

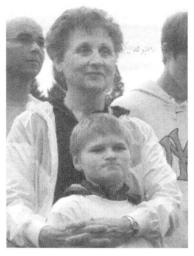

Youth Games 2011 Conrad and
his Grandma Jean Blumenauer

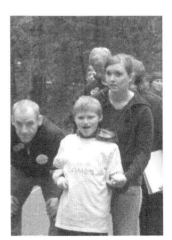

Youth Games 2011 Conrad
getting ready to run on
the track at Nike with
his caregiver Brittany

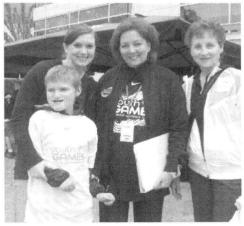

Youth Games 2011 Conrad, Brittany,
Grandma Margie and Grandma Jean

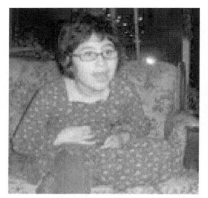

Priya Anand daughter
to Nicholette Anand

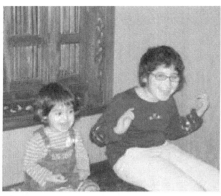

Priya Anand and her sister Seraphina

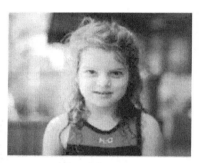

Sarah hergott

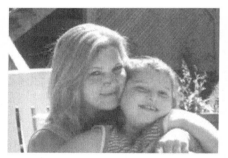

Sarah with her mom Leanne

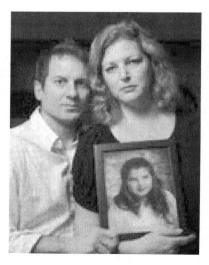

Paul and Leanne Hergott

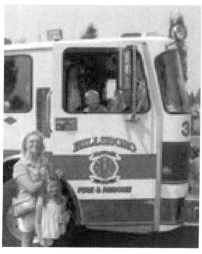

Adam Sprow

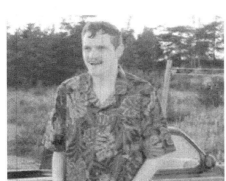

Graham Drover

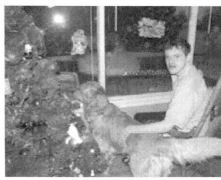

Graham Drover

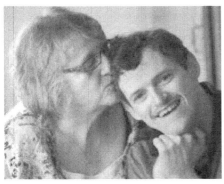

Graham and his mom Louise

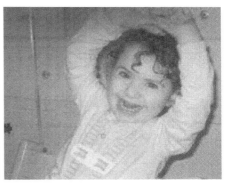

Ava Carlasarre

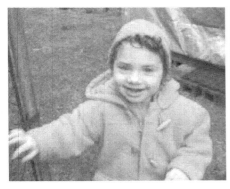

Ava Carlasarre

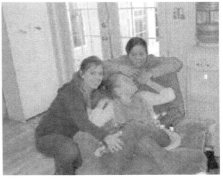

Patricia Schiffelers with two
of her amazing caregivers

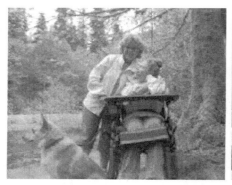

Patricia and her mother Christa

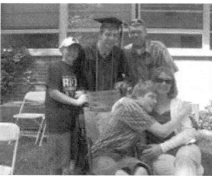

Sam Hickey and his family

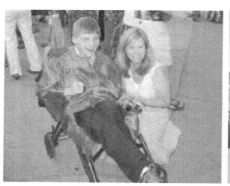

Sam Hickey at his graduation

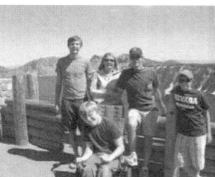

Sam Hickey and his family

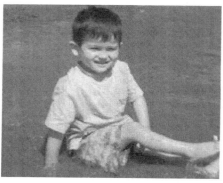

Elijah Humphries

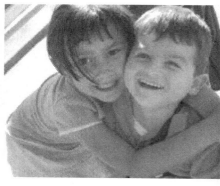

Elijah with his sister Francesca

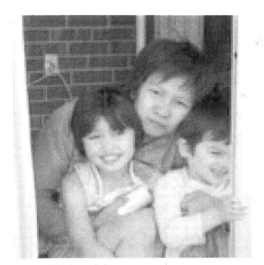

Elijah with his mom and sister

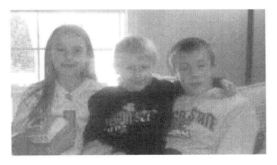

Joseph Hill with his sister Lauren
and his brother Nolan

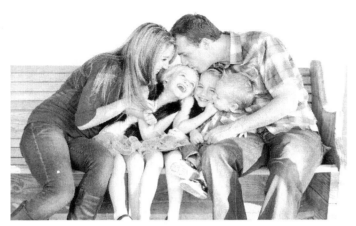

Kiley Joy and her family.

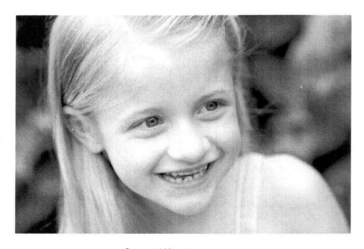

Sweet Kiley Joy.

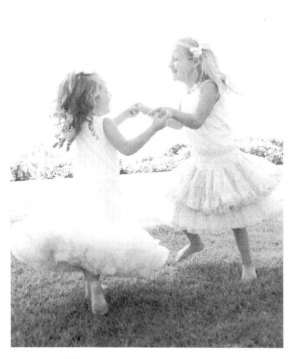

Kiley Joy dancing with her sister.

58126066R00143

Made in the USA
Lexington, KY
02 December 2016